BENNY HINN MINISTRIES PRESENTS

Fruits, Vegetables, & Herbs

FOR ENERGY, WELLNESS, AND POWER!

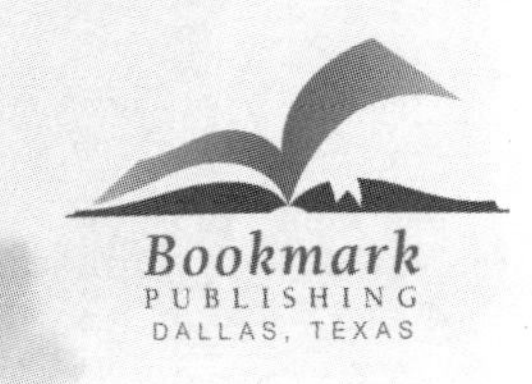

FRUITS, VEGETABLES, AND HERBS FOR ENERGY, WELLNESS, AND POWER!

Published by Bookmark Publishing
Dallas, Texas

Unless otherwise indicated, all Scripture quotations are taken from the *King James Version* of the Bible.

This information is not intended to replace the advice of physicians or nutritional professionals. Always consult your medical practitioner before making major changes in your diet or lifestyle.

ISBN: 1-59024-305-6

Printed in the United States of America.

10 9 8 7 6 5 4 3 2 1

www.BennyHinn.org

Contents

1

Fruits, Vegetables, and Herbs for a Healthy Lifestyle

So God created man in his own image, in the image of God created he him; male and female created he them. And God blessed them, and God said unto them, Be fruitful, and multiply, and replenish the earth, and subdue it: and have dominion over the fish of the sea, and over the fowl of the air, and over every living thing that moveth upon the earth.

—Genesis 1:27-28

God created Adam and Eve in the midst of the Garden of Eden, filled with life-giving bounty: "*And God said, Behold, I have given you every herb bearing seed, which is upon the face of all the earth, and every tree, in the which is the fruit of a tree yielding seed; to you it shall be for meat*" (Genesis 1:29).

Isn't it interesting that we often overlook the fact that God placed Adam and Eve in a garden—a paradise of fruits, vegetables, and herbs?

Today's leading nutrition researchers tell us why: Diets rich in fruits, vegetables, and herbs help us in so many ways by reducing the risk of cancer, heart disease, and other chronic challenges, meanwhile providing essential vitamins and minerals, fiber, and other substances that are important for good health.

Fruits, vegetables, and herbs are gifts from God, good for us and provided in abundance around the globe. These miracle foods were given by God for a specific purpose—optimum health and wellness—and they should be a large part of everyone's balanced and healthy eating plan.

Sadly, people today continue to stray increasingly from God's life-giving garden that He continues to provide. Studies, in fact, show that 90 percent of us are not eating nearly enough fruits, vegetables, and herbs! The results of that lack are obvious—obesity is epidemic and diseases related to nutritional imbalance continue to skyrocket.

Are you looking for a brighter future? Do you wish you could somehow eat healthier every day in the midst of your fast-paced, high-stress, snack-filled, fast-food, on-the-go world?

Fruits, Vegetables & Herbs for Energy, Wellness, & Power is filled with simple, informative, and easy ways to fill your life with God's natural bounty from His garden. No matter where you live, what your age, your lifestyle, or your cultural background, this book will help you discover quick, delicious, and convenient ways to eat more like our Creator designed you to eat with foods that can help keep you healthy throughout the years.

Eating fruits, vegetables, and herbs every day can help you in so many ways:

- Satisfying your body's need for vital vitamins and minerals
- Providing needed nutrition to sustain and restore your organs, tissue, bones, muscles, and skin
- Aiding with weight loss
- Bolstering your immune system
- Lowering your disease rates
- Thwarting the risk of cancer and diabetes
- Reducing cholesterol levels
- Fighting infection
- Preventing fatty accumulation in blood vessels that leads to heart disease
- Boosting your energy levels throughout the day

- Enriching your life and lifestyle, regardless of your age

Fruits, vegetables, and herbs have little or no cholesterol or fat. They are readily available, easy to prepare, comparatively economical, and delicious no matter how or when you serve them. There is a wide and interesting array from which to choose, regardless of where you live.

Combined with a healthy lifestyle, eating more fruits, vegetables, and herbs can be vital to your well-being. What could be better?

On the following pages you will learn the basics about fruits, vegetables, and herbs—their distinctive characteristics, health benefits, history, selection and shopping tips, storage, preparation, and ideas for serving.

God has provided fruits, vegetables, and herbs as a wonderful, life-giving bounty. This book takes away the mystery of eating from these tasty treasures for breakfast, lunch, dinner, and snacks as you develop a healthier lifestyle for you and your loved ones!

2

Fruits, Vegetables, and Herbs for Healthier Choices

And God said, Behold, I have given you every herb bearing seed, which is upon the face of all the earth, and every tree, in the which is the fruit of a tree yielding seed; to you it shall be for meat.

—Genesis 1:29

Quick! Think back to what you and your family ate today. How many servings of fruit did you eat? How many times did you include vegetables in meals or snacks? How often did you use herbs to enhance the flavors of the foods you prepared?

Yesterday? This past week?

Most government nutritional agencies around the globe recommend nutritional guidelines that include the following for each day:

- An emphasis on fruit (2 cups, or 2–4 servings), vegetables (2 1/2 cups, or 3–5 servings), herbs (used liberally to enhance your meals) every day
- Whole grains such as bread, cereal, rice, and pasta (6 ounces), with half of all grains

consumed to be whole grains, not highly processed breads, pastries, and sugary cereals

- Lean meats, poultry, fish, beans, eggs, nuts (5 1/2 ounces)
- Fat-free or low-fat milk and milk products such as yogurt and cheese (3 cups, or 2–3 servings)
- A small amount of saturated fats, trans fats, cholesterol, salt (sodium), and added sugars, all used sparingly
- 6–8 8-ounce glasses of water each day

Above all, nutrition experts agree that your food intake should stay within your daily caloric needs (2,000 is average each day; children need less, and some highly trained athletes need more). To lose weight, you need to reduce your caloric intake.

Learn the Food Groups

Even though this book will emphasize fruits, vegetables, and herbs, it is important to learn what

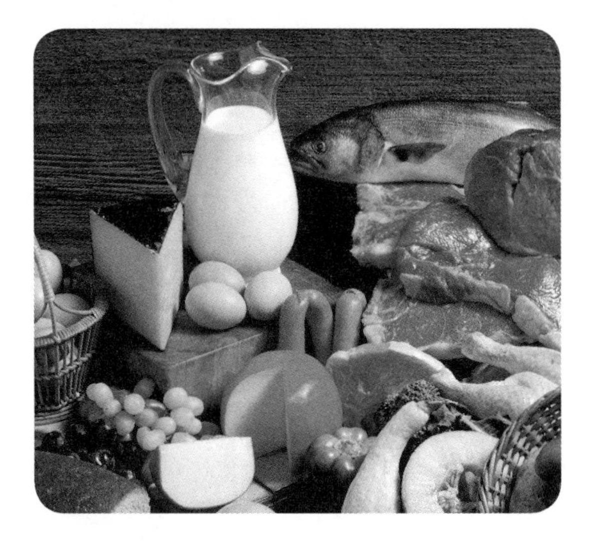

your ideal nutritional intake of food should be.

The following chart represents updated food guidelines, replacing the older food pyramid that was recognized for many years:

Anatomy of MyPyramid

One size doesn't fit all

USDA's new MyPyramid symbolizes a personalized approach to healthy eating and physical activity. The symbol has been designed to be simple. It has been developed to remind consumers to make healthy food choices and to be active every day. The different parts of the symbol are described below.

Activity

Activity is represented by the steps and the person climbing them, as a reminder of the importance of daily physical activity.

Moderation

Moderation is represented by the narrowing of each food group from bottom to top. The wider base stands for foods with little or no solid fats or added sugars. The narrower top area stands for foods containing more added sugars and solid fats. The more active you are, the more of these foods can fit into your diet.

Personalization

Personalization is shown by the person on the steps, the slogan, and the URL. Find the kinds and amounts of food to eat each day at MyPyramid.gov.

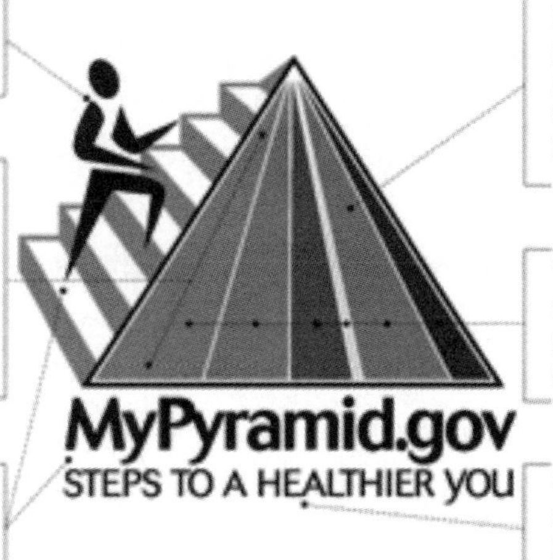

Proportionality

Proportionality is shown by the different widths of the food group bands. The widths suggest how much food a person should choose from each group. The widths are just a general guide, not exact proportions. Check the Web site for how much is right for you.

Variety

Variety is symbolized by the 6 color bands representing the 5 food groups of the Pyramid and oils. This illustrates that foods from all groups are needed each day for good health.

Gradual Improvement

Gradual improvement is encouraged by the slogan. It suggests that individuals can benefit from taking small steps to improve their diet and lifestyle each day.

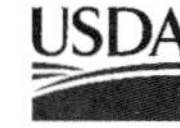

U.S. Department of Agriculture
Center for Nutrition Policy
and Promotion
April 2006 CNPP: 16

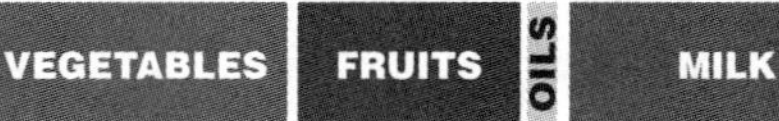

This is a general guide that lets you choose a variety-filled, balanced food plan that is right for you to maintain a healthy lifestyle.

Live a Healthier Lifestyle

The problem with most modern diets, however, is an overemphasis on starchy, sweet, and fat-laden meals and snacks, with a serious deficiency of fruits, vegetables, and herbs.

One of the main culprits in this deficiency is a food industry with a vested interest in producing foods that appeal to modern lifestyles and tastes. Quite frankly, they have provided an increasingly tempting array of foods that have helped us become addicted to starches, sugar, fat, and salt.

How bad is it?

The average American, for example, consumes 150–170 pounds of sugar each year! Americans spend $21 billion on candy alone.[1] Not surprisingly, 66 percent of American adults are overweight.[2] At least 40 million Americans are obese, with 3 million morbidly obese.

Sadly, this trend is exploding among children and young people. In 1982, only 4 percent of the nation's youngsters were considered overweight. By 1994 that number had risen to 16 percent. By 2001, the figure had soared to over 25 percent.[3] Unless something changes quickly, if adult statistics are an indication, the number of overweight children and young people will likely bulge to 50 percent or more during the next few years.

Recent studies by the U.S. Department of Agriculture, the National Cancer Institute, and the U.S. Center for Disease Control have revealed that a vast majority of Americans—fewer than one-third of adults—are not consuming the daily recommended amounts of fruits and vegetables suggested by the USDA.[4]

Specifically the CDC survey showed staggering statistics:

- Only 27 percent of adults ate vegetables three times a day, and only 33 percent ate fruit twice a day. (A serving size is considered to be a half cup for most fruits and vegetables, one cup for leafy greens.)
- Younger adults, ages 18–24, ate the fewest vegetables of all. Nearly four-fifths of that age category scraped the veggies to the side of their plates if they had vegetables on the plate at all.
- Senior citizens were more likely than others to follow Mom's advice to eat more veggies, yet only slightly more than a third of that group ate three or more servings each day.
- Seniors also consumed the most fruit, yet only 46 percent ate two or more servings of fruit daily.
- People ages 35–44 ate fruit the least, with fewer than 28 percent eating the recommended amount of fruit each day.[5]

Previous studies by these leading U.S. government agencies have clearly linked consumption of fruits and vegetables to a reduced risk of cancer and cardiovascular disease, and better weight management through the feeling of fullness and the decrease in the body's energy intake brought on by the foods.

In fact, the USDA cited these results as the primary reasons the agency switched from their famous "old" Food Guide Pyramid to the new MyPyramid system in 2005 (see page 7), which suggests an increased need for fruits and vegetables, and also offers recommendations on specific types of vegetables.

What about you? How can you start to eat a more balanced diet, especially with a greater emphasis on fruits, vegetables, and herbs?

Focus on Nutrient-Dense Foods

Fruits and vegetables, especially, are literally packed with nutrients, yet they are low in "extras" that just add calories. In other words, you get more bang for your proverbial buck! Most people could double or triple the daily intake of fruits and vegetables and still barely meet suggested minimums.

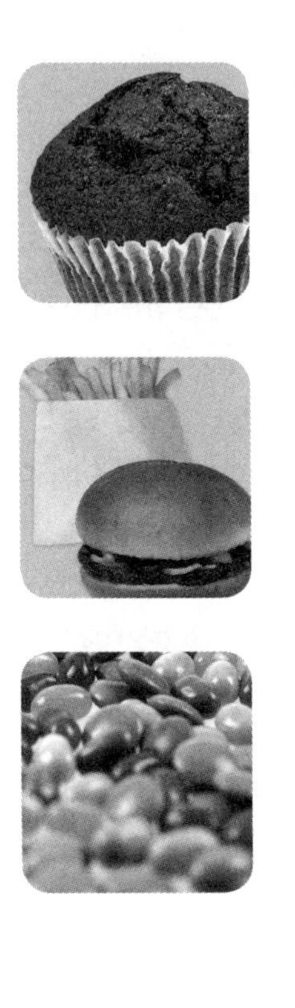

- Instead of a carbohydrate-heavy breakfast of a large muffin with butter (over 600 calories and at least 30 grams of fat), you can eat a large bowl of granola or shredded wheat with sliced bananas and skim milk (or soy milk), reducing the calories to less than 250 and the grams of fat to 2!
- Instead of a fast-food burger and fries (over 600 calories and over 30 grams of fat for lunch, opt for a large vegetable or fruit salad and lean meat sandwich on whole-grain bread, reducing the calories to less than 400 and grams of fat to 6.
- Instead of a midafternoon snack of a small handful of candy (over 200 calories) or potato chips (over 450 calories and 30 grams of fat), you could eat an entire plate of sliced veggies and low-fat dip (300 calories) or a plateful of fruit (approximately 200 calories and no fat).
- Instead of fried chicken and pasta with cream sauce (over

800 calories and nearly 50 grams of fat) for dinner, eat a hearty salad with a baked potato and lean portion of baked chicken or grilled salmon (400 calories and 5 grams of fat).

- Instead of pie a la mode (upwards to 900 calories and 45 grams of fat) for dessert, try a beautiful plate of fresh fruit (melon, berries, apples, or peaches) with a dip of sorbet or yogurt (under 300 calories).

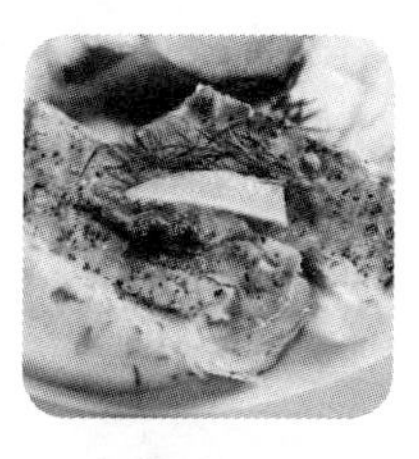

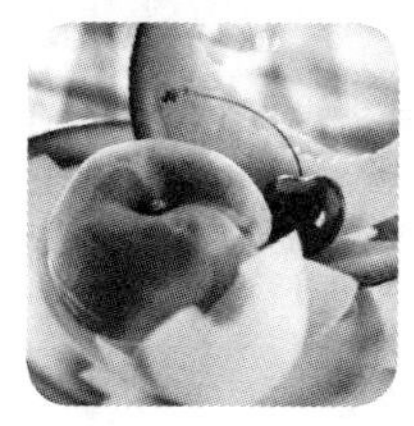

Watch Portion Sizes

As simple as it may seem, portion sizes matter greatly, regardless of what you eat. To eat healthier, it is important to focus on how much you eat. You can do this by weighing every bite of food, perhaps, but there is an easier way to be fairly accurate with your serving portions.

One easy rule of thumb relates to your actual thumb. Look at it now. A portion of food that size is approximately one ounce.

Now clench your fist. Fist sizes vary, of course, but the average clenched hand relates to approximately one cup of food.

With that in mind, since this is a book specifically dealing with fruits, vegetables, and herbs, remember that you should eat two fistfuls of fruit (2 cups or 2–4 servings) and 2 1/2 fistfuls of vegetables (2 1/2 cups, or 3–5 servings), plus the liberal use of herbs to enhance your meals every day. Generally, at least half of your plate at each snack or meal should be fruits and/or vegetables.

Generally, one serving of fruit might include:

- 1 medium-size apple, banana, or orange
- 1/2 cup diced mixed fruit salad
- 1/2 cup canned or frozen fruit
- 1/2 grapefruit
- 3/4 cup (6 ounces) fruit juice
- 1/4 cup raisins or other dried fruit
- 12 cherries or grapes

Generally, one serving of vegetables consists of:

- 1 cup raw vegetables or salad greens
- 1/2 cup chopped, sliced, or diced fresh vegetables
- 1/2 cup cooked, steamed, or grilled vegetables

Get Moving!

Physical activity can help you reach and keep a healthier weight, yet six out of ten Americans do not exercise at all![6] Regular physical activity is crucial for your overall health and well-being, and being active for 30–60 minutes on most days can help you actually gain more energy as you decrease your risk of disease, build strength and fitness, relax and reduce stress, and improve your sleep.

It is important to include activities that you enjoy and can easily fit into your daily routine, from walking your dog to working in the garden or riding your bicycle. It takes at least 60–90 days to develop a new habit, so it is important to start where you are and realize that it is important to commit to your daily exercise goal for a minimum of 2–3 months in order to get healthier for the long term.

Note: Always consult your physician before beginning any new activity or exercise program.

Track Food Intake and Physical Activity

Unless you find a way to measure your progress, you are not as likely to succeed with your new healthier lifestyle. Keep a notebook handy to follow your progress. Also, a great online resource for assessing your food intake and physical activity is www.mypyramidtracker.gov.

Change Your Lifestyle

Make changes to your lifestyle one meal at a time, one day at a time. The Bible clearly tells us, *"Do not despise these small beginnings, for the LORD rejoices to see the work begin"* (Zechariah 4:10, NLT). The most wonderful part of moving toward a healthier lifestyle is that you don't have to make drastic changes. Instead, you can take the following simple steps:

- Start with the top ten fruits (chapter 6), especially focusing on adding more fruit for breakfast and snacks.
- Keep everything simple with the top ten vegetables (chapter 7), adding a serving or two for lunch, snacks, and dinner.
- Use the top ten herbs (chapter 8) to add flavor to a dish at a time.
- Use the easy hints for adding fruits, vegetables, and herbs to breakfast (chapter 9), lunch (chapter 10), dinner (chapter 11), as well as snacks and desserts (chapter 12).

Most fruits, vegetables, and herbs are naturally low in both calories and fat. In addition, most contain good amounts of water and fiber to help give a feeling of fullness. When you combine these benefits with a more active lifestyle, eating greater amounts of fruits, vegetables, and herbs instead of high-calorie foods can help you control your weight and develop healthier habits.

In time, each of these "small beginnings" will change your life forever by giving you wellness, health, and power! Best of all, you begin to make healthier choices right now!

3

Fruits, Vegetables, and Herbs—Making the Transition

For the Lord *thy God bringeth thee into a good land, a land of brooks of water, of fountains and depths that spring out of valleys and hills; A land of wheat, and barley, and vines, and fig trees, and pomegranates; a land of oil olive, and honey.*

—Deuteronomy 8:7-8

Making the transition from the typical modern diet (fast food and starches) to a healthier lifestyle—including at least two fistfuls of fruit (2 cups or 2–4 servings), two and a half fistfuls of vegetables (2 1/2 cups, or 3–5 servings), and liberal amount of herbs to enhance your meals every day—means that at least half of your plate at each snack or meal should be fruits and vegetables.

Simply stated, that means that at least half of your time in the grocery store or market should be spent in the produce aisle (or fruits and vegetables section of the frozen foods aisle).

"Easier said than done!" you may be thinking.

It is easier said than done. That is why comparatively few people make the transition. That is why most people exit the supermarket with carts filled with starchy, prepared, sugar-filled foods and beverages.

You must make a choice to make the transition. You must continue making healthy choices. However, even "small beginnings" in time will change your life forever by giving you energy, wellness, and power! This is certainly true when it comes to planning your meals and shopping for the right kinds of foods.

Menu Planning

Planning ahead is the key to success! If you don't stock fruits, vegetables, and herbs in your kitchen, you will not have them available when you're hungry.

However, don't change your entire world in one gigantic leap. Make small changes at first. Stuffing your refrigerator with healthy foods will mean little unless you make plans to use what you purchase.

Don't leave things to chance. Sit down and sketch out a simple menu for several days. Make sure to include plenty of fruits, vegetables, and herbs in your plans—perhaps even use a highlighter to spotlight the healthy additions to your diet.

Search books and magazines for recipes that you and your family may enjoy. Keep an eye out for dishes that incorporate fruits, vegetables, and herbs. This helps you in making the transition toward healthier meals and snacks. New ideas and tastes can be both fun and nutritious!

Once you put together the menu for a few days, then simplify the foods into a shopping list that you can follow easily when you go through your neighborhood grocery store or farmers' market. Read your weekly newspaper food section for local grocery sales and menu ideas (some newspapers also offer nutritious recipes with these menus).

If possible, divide your list into sections—produce, breads and baked goods, canned goods, pastas, baking supplies, pet supplies, beverages, cleaning supplies, snacks, dairy, meats, frozen food—

that closely and conveniently follow the layout of your favorite supermarkets.

Shopping Guidelines

Here are several ways to plan your meals and shop to make sure you enjoy at least 2 cups (or 2–4 servings) of fruits, 2 1/2 cups (3–5 servings) of vegetables, and liberal amount of herbs every day without complicating your busy life:

- As mentioned, plan your shopping trips with the store's layout in mind, then keep your list handy and mark off each item as you place it in the cart. Research shows that buying from a list is more economical and avoids impulse purchases that you should avoid. This also helps keep things organized if you are a coupon clipper.
- Many stores have a convenient stack of weekly circulars with sale items, specials, and store coupons inside. Use them!
- Never go shopping when you are hungry! You have probably heard this before, but it is true. Research shows that people who shop hungry often buy foods that are high in sugar, fat, and calories, and low in nutrition.
- Spend more time in the produce aisles than anywhere else in the store or market. More delicious, unique, colorful, and exotic items are available than ever before, and this vast array can sometimes be overwhelming. Take your time. Use your senses—sight, smell, taste, and feel. Educate yourself. Many stores have nutrition, recipes, and serving suggestions with the fruits, vegetables, and herbs. Start by trying a new produce item each time you shop.
- Even though nearly every produce item is now available year round with refrigeration, storage, and shipping advancements, it still makes sense in so many ways to buy produce in peak season for better taste, quality, and price.

- Most produce departments have a wonderful selection of bagged salads, often with a variety of lettuces and other vegetables. These offer a wonderful opportunity to try different blends without having to purchase a mountain of different salad items.
- If your store has a buy-by-the-pound salad bar in the produce aisle or deli area, take advantage of the already-prepared raw vegetables and fruits that you have not tried before. You can buy as little or as much as you want to try.
- Many produce departments also have fresh bags of soup ingredients. Again, you don't have to decide what vegetables to buy. Everything is in the container. All you do when you get home is dump the items in a large pot and follow the instructions printed on the bag. It's easy, simple, and tastes so much better after the flavorful aromas fill your kitchen while stewing.
- Plan to add unusual or untried varieties of vegetables and fruits when you prepare soups, casseroles, and sauces—perhaps something as simple as grated carrots and zucchini to spaghetti sauce. This simple tip adds interesting color to your meals and can be an easy way to add more and more healthy items to your meals.
- Be sure to buy a few fresh herbs as you go through the produce aisles. Most markets sell small amounts to allow you to experiment with these flavor enhancers without breaking the bank. Chapter 8 of this book will help you learn more about ways to add more herbs to your meals.
- Be sure to stock up on healthy vegetable and fruit drinks, rather than caffeine-, chemical-, and sugar-laced soft drinks.

- Think of fruits for dessert and snacks as you wheel through the supermarket, rather than hitting the appealing aisles filled with chips, cookies, pastries, and ice creams.
- Read all labels. Note that the items are listed from the most to the least. Avoid sugars, chemicals, starches, fats, and high salt (sodium) content.
- Organic is generally better than bulk produce that may have been sprayed with insecticides. Fresh is generally better than prepared, canned, or packaged foods.
- Don't hesitate to purchase frozen fruits and vegetables, which are usually frozen at the peak of ripeness, but avoid produce frozen with high sugar or sodium content.
- Look for loss-leader specials. Many times supermarkets offer buy-one-get-one-free for advertising purposes. The savings can be substantial if it is a bag of potatoes, apples, carrots, or oranges. Take advantage of these specials, and be sure to stock up only on produce that will not spoil quickly.
- Take stock of your produce inventory before making your next shopping trip. See what fruits, vegetables, and herbs are lurking behind other items in the refrigerator and use them first, avoiding waste.
- Most produce does not have a long shelf life, so only purchase what you can realistically store and use. Grocery stores get fresh produce regularly, so you can always have fresh items available by planning your shopping trips wisely.
- If possible, get to know the produce people at each grocery store or market where you shop. They can often offer a wealth of information about produce selections and variety, what is in season, preparation tips, and cost-cutting suggestions.

- If you live more than 20–30 minutes away from your supermarket, think about placing frozen and easy-to-spoil items in an ice-filled cooler in the backseat or trunk of your vehicle.

One final note concerning shopping: Be careful as you prepare to check out. The stores don't call them impulse items for nothing. You're hungry. You're tired. Your kids are begging for goodies lined up and down the checkout lane. Learn to focus on the colorful fruits, vegetables, and herbs in your cart, rather than the candy bars screaming your name!

Think about how wonderful you will feel after eating healthy foods and snacks, as opposed to the sugar high you get from "just a little nibble" of those packs of munchies stacked on the shelves within easy reach.

Mercifully, many stores now stock ice cold bottled water in the convenient coolers of soft drinks next to the checkout lanes. Grab a bottle of H_2O if you have to buy something impulsively before exiting with your items, then mentally pat yourself on the back for avoiding the hundreds, perhaps thousands of calories you might have gobbled down on the ride home.

Nobody said it would be easy to transition into a new, healthy lifestyle; however, with each positive choice you make, every small beginning, the decisions become easier as you begin to have more energy, become healthier, and feel better about yourself.

Keep It Simple

So many people tend to put off eating more fruits, vegetables, and herbs because it all seems so complicated. You can greatly improve success as you make the transition to a healthier eating lifestyle by choosing to keep things very simple.

Start at your own pace. Experiment with new fruits, vegetables, and herbs to discover what you like and don't like. Educate yourself. Stay open to the possibilities.

Most of all, enjoy the transition!

4

Fruits, Vegetables, and Herbs—Wellness Guidelines

I will praise thee; for I am fearfully and wonderfully made: marvellous are thy works; and that my soul knoweth right well.

—Psalm 139:14

God's people should be healthy people. His Word has given explicit guidelines to follow which promise health and healing in every area of our lives.

Just for starters, the human body was designed perfectly from an incredibly complex blueprint. In fact, the more science learns about the human makeup, the more complicated and complex it becomes. The body's structure—from the crown of your head to the soles of your feet—is an absolutely awesome miracle of precision and meticulousness that could have only been designed by a loving Creator.

Your major organs alone—including the heart, lungs, brain, eyes, stomach, spleen, bones, pancreas, kidneys, liver, intestines, skin (the largest human organ), reproductive organs, and bladder—perform such amazing functions that entire medical libraries throughout the world are filled with volumes that attempt to explain each one adequately. Those libraries are constantly being updated with new findings that continue to amaze researchers.

Much of the newest research points to the fact that humans are designed to primarily digest plant foods. Quoting from Michael Murray, N.D., in his book, *The Encyclopedia of Healing Foods*:

> Specifically, our teeth are composed of twenty molars, which are perfect for crushing and grinding plant foods, along with eight front incisors, which are well suited for biting into fruits and vegetables. Only our front four canine teeth are designed for meat eating, and our jaws swing both vertically to tear and laterally to crush, while carnivores' jaws swing only vertically. Additional evidence that supports the human body's preference for plant foods is the long length of the human intestinal tract. Carnivores typically have a short bowel, while herbivores have a bowel length proportionally comparable to humans.[1]

There is a great variety of opinions about the biblical diet. Do we eat meat (as did Abraham, Isaac, Jacob, Moses, and David, for example)? Do we eat fish, as Jesus did when He performed the miracle feeding of the five thousand, when He ate with His disciples during the Last Supper and after the Resurrection? Or do we eat only vegetables, fruits, and herbs, as many Christians believe—running the gamut from lacto vegetarians, who eat dairy products, ovo vegetarians, who don't eat dairy products but do eat eggs, semivegetarians, who don't eat red meat but do eat fish, eggs, and dairy products, to vegans, who totally depend upon plant-based food for nutrition.

Regardless of how you believe concerning fish and meat, we do know that the oldest diet known to creation was established by God Himself in the Garden of Eden: "*And God said, 'See, I have given you every herb that yields seed which is on the face of all the earth, and every tree whose fruit yields seed; to you it shall be for food'"* (Genesis 1:29, NKJV).

The two earliest sources of nutrition for mankind were herbs and fruits. Fruits are fairly self-explanatory. Herbs, however, used in this context as a Hebrew word, included a wide variety of foods including grasses (barley, wheat, rice, and more), berry plants, vegetables, legumes, beans, herbs, and spices. Olives and grapes are also often mentioned positively in the Bible.

So whether you eat meat or not, it is apparent that the ideal has always been to include as many fruits, vegetables, and herbs as possible. Dr. Don Colbert says, "These items should form the largest part of your diet. At least 35 percent of our food intake should be from fruits and vegetables."[2]

Dr. Colbert also writes:

> Healing and divine health are God's perfect will for mankind. God created Adam as a healthy being—a perfect act of creation. We find no record of sickness until Adam chose to disobey God. Sickness and disease entered the human race because of Adam's sin. God's plan was that he would enjoy divine health.[3]

In the Garden of Eden, we have a template of the perfect foods which God created for man. Then during the Exodus, we have additional instructions concerning a healthy lifestyle:

> *If thou wilt diligently hearken to the voice of the* LORD *thy God, and wilt do that which is right in his sight, and wilt give ear to his commandments, and keep all his statutes, I will put none of these diseases upon thee, which I have brought upon the Egyptians: for I am the* LORD *that healeth thee.* (Exodus 15:26)

We can claim this promise as we obey the LORD, eat nutritionally balanced meals, exercise, and live wholesomely. The LORD later gave more complete dietary instructions to the Israelites:

For the LORD thy God bringeth thee into a good land, a land of brooks of water, of fountains and depths that spring out of valleys and hills; A land of wheat, and barley, and vines, and fig trees, and pomegranates; a land of oil olive, and honey; A land wherein thou shalt eat bread without scarceness, thou shalt not lack any thing in it; a land whose stones are iron, and out of whose hills thou mayest dig brass. (Deuteronomy 8:7-9)

We must be wise as we follow God's directions and guidance in every area of our lives. Again, no matter what you believe in terms of eating meat, poultry, fish, and dairy products, it is apparent we were designed with an ideal nutritional intake that focuses largely on plant-based foods. It worked perfectly in the Garden of Eden and later in the Promised Land. We can therefore assume that we can reap the same benefits as we partake of the best foods.

A biblically sound diet of lots of fruits, vegetables, and herbs can help keep your heart healthy, prevent diabetes and other diseases, and help you feel and look younger.

Disease Prevention

Diseases fill our world—from heart problems to diabetes, cancer, and an ever-increasing dictionary of new medical challenges—yet we see in Genesis that humans were brought into a perfect world, perfectly designed by the Creator for maximum health.

What happened?

The Bible offers the way to live under God's pattern for health and abundant blessings. As we have seen in Exodus 15, God even promised that His people would suffer "none of these diseases" if they would only follow His guidelines.

What happened is what continues to take place. We follow man's ideas instead of the Creator's.

Dr. Rex Russell, in his book *What the Bible Says About Healthy Living*, offers this clear-cut directive:

"Wise people will follow the Divine Design for health. If we were all wise, we would rarely need doctors.... We would all put ourselves under the care of Him who brought Israel out of Egypt, having 'not one feeble person among their tribes' (Psalm 105:37)." [4]

A Healthy Heart

More money is spent treating heart disease than any other illness. We know that heart disease is the leading cause of death in the United States, claiming hundreds of thousands of lives each year.

According to the Center for Disease Control and American Heart Association statistics, heart disease and strokes—leading components of cardiovascular disease—are the first and third leading causes of death in the United States.[5] Additionally, according to the same reports:

- Heart disease and strokes accounted for nearly 40 percent of all deaths.
- About 70 million Americans (almost one-fourth of the population) have some form of cardiovascular disease, which is responsible for more than 6 million hospitalizations each year.
- About 90 percent of middle-aged Americans will develop high blood pressure in their lifetime, and nearly 70 percent of those who have it now do not have it under control.

The prevention and control of the major risk factors for heart disease and stroke are critical to achieving a heart-healthy and stroke-free lifestyle. Individuals can reduce their chance of developing heart disease by exercising regularly, maintaining healthy eating habits and weight, avoiding tobacco use, and monitoring cholesterol and blood pressure levels.

What part can eating more fruits, vegetables, and herbs play in helping you have a healthier heart?

Writes Dr. Don Colbert: "People in underdeveloped nations who cannot afford to eat steak, butter, and fatty foods experience very little heart disease. Their so-called poverty diets consist of healthy fruits, grains, and vegetables."[6]

Prevention of heart disease should begin during your childhood and continue through your life, but you can begin your healthy heart program today. Reducing your LDL cholesterol by 50 points, for example, can reduce the risk of a heart attack or stroke by as much as 50 percent, so the sooner you get started, the better!

One of the best ways is to substantially reduce saturated fat intake (which includes cutting back on red meats, high-fat dairy products, sweets, and high-carbohydrate foods), take advantage of monounsaturated fats which help reduce LDL cholesterol (including olive oil, canola oil, avocados, nuts, seeds), and dramatically increase fruits, vegetables, and herbs—great sources of vitamins and minerals that are essential to your health.

Dr. Paavo Airola, long considered a leading voice in the therapeutic uses of natural foods, points especially to a greater intake of vegetables such as carrots, beets, celery, asparagus, garlic, and onions, and fruits such as red grapes, black currants, rose hips, and blueberries.[7]

Diabetes

According to the American Diabetes Association, we are in the midst of an epidemic with 20.8 million children and adults in the United States, or 7 percent of the population, with diabetes. While an estimated 14.6 million have been diagnosed with type 1 or type 2 diabetes, unfortunately, 6.2 million people (or nearly one-third) are unaware that they have the disease.[8]

In addition, there are 54 million Americans who have prediabetes, a condition that occurs when a person's blood glucose levels are higher than normal but not high enough for a diagnosis of type 2 diabetes.

Diabetes is a disease in which the body does not produce or properly use insulin, a hormone needed to convert sugar, starches, and other food into energy. Both genetics and environmental factors such as obesity, lack of proper diet, and lack of exercise appear to play roles.

Obesity and diabetes are fearsome teammates, since the more fat cells you have, the more difficult it is to get glucose (sugar) to the muscles. This condition known as "insulin resistance" keeps sugar from the muscles, causing it to stay longer in the bloodstream, which results in a number of problems.

Most people with diabetes have increased health problems, including arteriosclerosis (hardening of the arteries), blindness, kidney failure, neuropathy (nerve damage and loss of feeling, especially in feet and hands), and amputation. High blood pressure and cholesterol, combined with diabetes, mean that more than 65 percent of people with diabetes die from heart disease or stroke.

However, by managing diabetes, high blood pressure, and cholesterol, people with diabetes can reduce risks. Reversing the trends that lead to diabetes should include not only increased activity, but also a healthier diet of certain fruits, nearly all vegetables, and herbs that are filled with fiber, antioxidants, minerals, vitamins, and phytonutrients.

According to Dr. Paavo Airola, a proponent of natural therapies for the treatment of sickness and disease, offers an interesting point: "Diabetics have a tendency for overacidity because of slowed down protein and fat metabolism. Therefore, the diet should be alkaline, with emphasis on alkaline foods: vegetables, fruits...cucumbers, stringbeans, Jerusalem artichokes, and garlic."[9]

Cancer

Long considered a "prosperity" disease, cancer is a term for diseases in which abnormal cells divide without control and often invade other tissues, spreading to other parts of the body through the blood and lymph systems. There are more than a hundred different types of cancer.

In the U.S. and other developed countries, cancer is presently responsible for about 25 percent of all deaths.[10] In fact, cancer has surpassed heart disease as the leading cause of death for people younger than eighty-five since 1999.[11]

There are many contributing factors for the dramatic prevalence of this disease, and huge amounts of money are spent each year seeking new ways to prevent this horrible disease.

The general consensus shows that modern diets greatly increase the risk of developing cancer. Study after study of people around the world with higher intakes of plant-based foods show a marked decrease in cancer. Eating phytonutrient- and antioxidant-filled fruits (such as raspberries, grapefruit, grapes, oranges, cantaloupe, and tomatoes), vegetables (including broccoli, cabbage, cauliflower, garlic, onions, sweet potatoes), and herbs (including ginseng, golden seal, dandelion root) are often mentioned as helpful in preventing cancer, especially as you limit your fat intake.

Aging Gracefully

Your health and vitality depend upon a weblike association of many different components such as nutrition, stress, biochemistry, genes, and fitness. Certain things not only keep you from aging rapidly, but actually turn back the clock.

In other words, your life and health depend upon factors largely under your own control. While this is by no means an exhaustive list, here are several practical ways you can take control of aging:

- Be aware of your genetic weaknesses and strengths. You can't choose your genes, of course, but you can be alert to tendencies that run in your family and seek to overcome those traits. Get tested more often for conditions with a higher risk.
- Change your future! Just because someone

in your family died from a heart attack when they were 55 or 65 or 105 doesn't mean that you have to fall into a chasm of self-fulfilling prophecy. Seek medical guidance on how to overcome genetic traits, then change what you can.

- Realize that time is on your side. The life-expectancy numbers are rising by the year. Modern medicine continues to unravel many secrets of illness and genetic challenges. Preventative medicine is exploding with new solutions to age-old questions. Seek out information, and learn what works for you.
- Resolve to get more fit and healthy. Regardless of where you are right now—good, bad, or in-between—you can get better. Study after study of people from all age groups—even those in their nineties—show that those who follow a program of health and fitness tend to live longer and with a better quality of life.

Most importantly, eat to get younger. Dr. Michael Roizen, in his powerful book *The RealAge Diet*, says that you can add years to your life (and life to your years) by doing something as simple as eating more fresh fruits and vegetables, whole-grain breads, beans, and brown rice. He and coauthor Dr. John La Puma show how they have helped many reverse aging by changing lifestyle choices. They name fifty-one age-buster foods.[12]

Dr. Paavo Airola, cited earlier for his natural therapies, points to the need for anti-aging vitamins B and E, along with lots of vegetables and fruit juices (including pineapple, papaya, lemon, lime, and apricot), as well as herbs such as ginseng, gotu-kola, garlic, and sarsaparilla.[13] Other fruits (including blueberries, citrus, cherries, watermelon, and tomatoes) and vegetables (including kale and spinach) are often cited by nutritional professionals as filled with beneficial antiaging antioxidants to help boost memory, cancer protection, heart health, arthritis, and memory.

The point is this: Fruits, vegetables, and herbs help you look and feel better. The better you look and feel, the better you feel about yourself. As a result, you perform better and others respond to you more positively. It is a life-giving, positive cycle that anyone can achieve!

Think young! Seek God's guidance in your life, no matter how many birthday candles you get to blow out each year. Without the Lord in your life, you are running in circles with no end in sight. With Him, you have meaning and direction.

Remember, you are responsible for you. Free choice is a tremendous gift from God, but it is also a life-or-death challenge. It is up to you to make changes in your lifestyle and environment that will contribute to better health and turn back the clock.

5

Fruits, Vegetables, and Herbs —Vitamins, Minerals, and Nutritional Values

My people are destroyed for lack of knowledge.

—Hosea 4:6

God created good foods to provide wellness. Not taking care of the body with nutritionally balanced meals and exercise means that we will suffer the physical and emotional consequences of poor health. However, eating and living the way God intended brings vitality and health.

Therefore, the main reason why you should include more fruits, vegetables, and herbs is because they are chockfull of vitamins and minerals which help your body work properly in many ways:

- Vitamins fall into two categories: fat soluble and water soluble. The fat-soluble vitamins (A, D, E, and K) dissolve in fat and can be stored in your body. The water-soluble vitamins (C and the B-complex vitamins including vitamins B_6, B_{12}, niacin, riboflavin, and folate) need to dissolve in water before your body can absorb them and cannot be stored. Therefore, you especially need a fresh supply of water-soluble vitamins.

- Minerals are inorganic elements that come from the soil and water and are absorbed by plants or eaten by animals, whereas vitamins are organic substances from plants or animals. Your body needs larger amounts of some minerals, such as calcium, to grow and stay healthy. Other minerals like chromium, copper, iodine, iron, selenium, and zinc are called trace minerals because you need only very small amounts of them each day.

Although you get vitamins and minerals from the foods you eat every day, some foods—especially fruits, vegetables, and herbs—have more beneficial vitamins and minerals than others, as the following chart outlines:

Nutrient	Functions and Benefits	Food Sources	DRI (Daily Recommended Intake)[1]
FAT-SOLUBLE VITAMINS—natural substances found in plants and animals. Your body has to use bile acids to absorb fat-soluble vitamins. Once these vitamins are absorbed, your body stores them in body fat. When you need them, your body uses them from where they are stored. Eating fats or oils that are not digested can cause shortages of fat-soluble vitamins.			

Abbreviations: IU=International Units; mg=milligrams; mcg=micrograms

Nutrient	Functions and Benefits	Food Sources	DRI (Daily Recommended Intake)
Vitamin A	Helps maintain good vision (necessary for night vision), promotes growth and repair of body tissues, bone formation, healthy skin, and hair. Essential for immune system and resistance to infections. Supports growth and repair of body tissue. Also maintains integrity of white and red blood cells. Beta carotene, which is converted to vitamin A in the body, serves as an antioxidant, which can help protect against cancer, heart disease, and cataracts. Vitamin A deficiency can lead to night blindness, reduced hair growth in children, dry eyes, lowered resistance to infection, dry skin.	Beta carotene and other carotenoids are found in green leafy vegetables (kale, broccoli, spinach, collard and turnip greens, parsley, and escarole. Yellow vegetables that help provide vitamin A include carrots, pumpkin, sweet potatoes, and winter squash. Yellow and orange fruits with vitamin A include papaya, apricots, mango, and cantaloupe. Also found in milk, eggs, meat, fish liver oils.	3, 000 IU Some nutritional professionals recommend as much as 5,000 IU.

Nutrient	Functions and Benefits	Food Sources	DRI (Daily Recommended Intake)
Vitamin D	Known as the "sunshine vitamin." Helps build and maintain healthy teeth and bones. Enhances calcium absorption. Vitamin D deficiency can lead to rickets in children and bone softening and osteoporosis in adults.	Exposure to sun, also found in dairy products, egg yolks, fish liver oils, tuna, mackerel, herring, sardines, oysters, yeast.	Men: 500 IU Women: 400 IU
Vitamin E	This antioxidant helps form red blood cells, muscles, and other tissue. Helps to reduce the risk of certain forms of cancer and prevent anemia. Vitamin E deficiency can lead to degeneration in the coronary system (which can lead to strokes and heart disease). Prolonged deficiency can cause reproductive, muscular, and nerve disorders, as well as weakened red blood cells.	Found primarily in vegetable oils (corn, cottonseed, soybean), rice, nuts, avocados, eggs, whole grain cereals, and wheat germ. Green leafy vegetables are also a great natural source of vitamin E.	15 mg Some nutritional professionals suggest 30–200 mg per day, and even higher for therapeutic doses.

Nutrient	Functions and Benefits	Food Sources	DRI (Daily Recommended Intake)
Vitamin K	The "anti-hemorrhaging" vitamin, K is essential for blood clotting, bone health, and normal liver function. It is also important to vitality and longevity. A vitamin K deficiency can cause hemorrhages anywhere in the body, premature aging, and lowered vitality.	Green, leafy vegetables are the best source, as well as soybean oil, egg yolks, cow's milk, and liver. Vitamin K is also manufactured by bacteria in healthy intestines.	Not determined. Some nutritional professionals suggest as much as 80 mcg (men) 65 mcg (women)

Nutrient	Functions and Benefits	Food Sources	DRI (Daily Recommended Intake)
WATER-SOLUBLE VITAMINS—natural substances found in plants and animals. Water-soluble vitamins are easily absorbed by your body. Unlike fat-soluble vitamins, they don't have to be absorbed using bile acids. Your body doesn't store large amounts of water-soluble vitamins. The water-soluble vitamins you don't need are removed by your kidneys and flushed out of your body.			
Vitamin B_1 Thiamine	A great antiaging vitamin, B_1 helps metabolize carbohydrates and proteins, maintains appetite and normal digestion, is essential for nerve tissue function, helps maintain a normal red blood count, improves circulation, prevents fatigue, and increases stamina. A vitamin B_1 deficiency can lead to muscular weakness, a lack of appetite, irritability, diabetes, depression, and nervous exhaustion.	Found in many foods: whole grain cereals, brown rice, peas, sunflower seeds, beans, peanuts, legumes, brewer's yeast, and wheat germ. A deficiency of Vitamin B_1 can be caused by excess alcohol, sugar, and overly produced, highly refined foods.	1.2 mg (men) 1.1 mg (women)

Nutrient	Functions and Benefits	Food Sources	DRI (Daily Recommended Intake)
Vitamin B_2 Riboflavin	Essential for the release of energy and the proper function of the nervous system, vitamin B_2 is vital for growth, general health, eyes, skin, hair, and nails. It helps the body regulate energy, break down amino acids, and regulate hormones. It is important in the formation of red blood cells. Research shows that B_2 also helps protect against cataracts. Supports cellular breathing. Prevents red, cracked lips and burning tongue. May help with high lactate or lactic acidosis. A B_2 deficiency can result in inflammation in the mouth, itching and burning of the eyes, eczema, ulcers, dull or oily hair, premature wrinkles, and anemia.	Milk, cheese, whole grains, egg whites, leafy vegetables such as spinach, liver, lean meat, fish, wheat germ, yogurt, brewer's yeast, almonds, and mushrooms are all reported to be good sources.	1.3 mg (men) 1.1 mg (women) Some nutritional professionals promote doses as high as 25–50 mg per day.

Nutrient	Functions and Benefits	Food Sources	DRI (Daily Recommended Intake)
Vitamin B_3 Niacin, nicotinic acid Niacinamide is similar in effect but does not cause skin flushing that often occurs when niacin is taken.	Important for proper circulation, protein, and carbohydrate metabolism, fat synthesis, healthy skin, respiration, digestive system, and may help manage cholesterol. Deficiencies include canker sores, skin problems, insomnia, digestive disorders, depression, and other nervous disorders.	Brewer's yeast, legumes, whole grains, peanuts, Nuts, sunflower seeds, green vegetables, liver, brown rice, lean meat, chicken, salmon, and tuna	Niacin: 16 mg (men) 14 mg (women) Supplements at a much higher dose are sometimes used as a therapy for high LDL cholesterol, but can cause itching and flushing. This should be done only with a physician's supervision. You can also take niacinamide, a nonitchy, no-flush supplement form of B_3. Some nutritional professionals advise as high as 250 mg a day.

Nutrient	Functions and Benefits	Food Sources	DRI (Daily Recommended Intake)
Vitamin B_5 Panthothenic acid	Helps body metabolize carbohydrates, fats, and make steroids. Wards off infections and speeds recovery from ill health. Needed to manufacture adrenal chemicals and chemicals that regulate nerve function. Offsets deficiency-related dermatitis and “burning foot” syndrome. Can help prevent premature aging, especially wrinkles. Deficiencies, while somewhat uncommon due to its widespread availability in foods, can include chronic fatigue, depression, muscular weakness, skin disorders, and allergies.	Abundant in legumes, avocados, soybeans, whole grains, brewer’s yeast, green vegetables, peas and beans, peanuts, eggs, chicken, and liver.	2.5 mg (men and women) 10 mg is included in most B vitamin complex supplements. Some natural health practitioners recommend as high as 30–50 mg a day.

Nutrient	Functions and Benefits	Food Sources	DRI (Daily Recommended Intake)
Vitamin B_6 Pyridoxine, pyridoxal, other forms	Necessary for protein and carbohydrate metabolism. Helps form healthy red blood cells. Promotes brain and nerve function. Deficiencies include skin and nerve disorders, sore mouth and lips, insomnia, premature senility, and anemia.	Bananas, avocados, cantaloupe, cabbage, green leafy vegetables, green peppers, carrots, pecans, chicken, fish, pork, liver, eggs, brown rice, soybeans, oats, and whole wheat. Raw vegetables and fruit provide more B6 than cooked.	1.3–2.0 mg Some nutrition professionals recommend as high as 250 mg per day, especially if taken in a B complex supplement.

Nutrient	Functions and Benefits	Food Sources	DRI (Daily Recommended Intake)
Vitamin B_{12} Cobalamin	Sometimes called the "red vitamin" because it aids in red blood cell health and development, promotes growth in children, involved in many of the body's metabolic and enzymatic processes, builds genetic materials, and is used in management of neuropathy. We store 2–5 mcg of vitamin B_{12} and only excrete a very small fraction of this each day. Nevertheless, over time, a vitamin B_{12} deficiency can develop if stores are not replenished from the diet or from supplements.[2] Deficiencies in vitamin B_{12} can result in poor growth in children, chronic fatigue, numbness or stiffness, low mental energy, nerve damage.	Liver, kidney, dairy, eggs. Tempeh, miso, sea vegetables, and other plant foods are sometimes reported to contain vitamin B_{12}. Since vitamin B_{12} is present in vegetables and fruits only in small amounts, vegans and vegetarians often use brewer's yeast or take supplements or injections. B_{12} is synthesized by intestinal bacteria. Many people use acidophilus supplements to help maintain intestinal flora.	2.4 mcg Therapeutic doses of as much as 50–100 mcg are sometimes recommended. Vitamin B_{12} is more complicated than other B vitamins. The body can make and recycle some B_{12} from what comes in, but absorption of this vitamin can be disrupted in both the stomach and the intestines. Many who are deficient must take B_{12} injections.

Nutrient	Functions and Benefits	Food Sources	DRI (Daily Recommended Intake)
Biotin (Sometimes called vitamin H)	Needed for fat, carbohydrate, glucose, and amino acid metabolism, as well as overall proper body chemistry. Deficiency can result in fatigue, hair loss, skin disorders, heart abnormalities, lung infections, depression, and drowsiness.	Brewer's yeast is the best source; also found in cauliflower, soybeans, brown rice, peanut butter, nuts, eggs, milk, cheese, kidney, and liver.	30–150 mcg Some nutritional professionals recommend as much as 300 mcg for deficiencies. B complex vitamins often contain 30– 100 mcg of biotin.

Nutrient	Functions and Benefits	Food Sources	DRI (Daily Recommended Intake)
Vitamin C Ascorbic acid	Essential for healthy function of all glands and organs, C is necessary for wound healing, bone fractures, and resistance to infections. Strengthens connective tissues and blood vessels. Helps prevent and cure the common cold. It is a general detoxicant and protects against all forms of stress. Also aids in the absorption of iron. Deficiencies of vitamin C can lead to muscle weakness, easy bruising, tooth decay, premature aging, thyroid insufficiency, and lowered resistance to all infections.	Abundant in most fresh fruits (especially citrus) and vegetables. It is especially rich in rose hips, black currants, strawberries, apples, persimmons, guavas, acerola cherries, potatoes, cabbage, broccoli, tomatoes, turnip greens, and green bell peppers.	90 mg (men) 75 mg (women) Therapeutic recommendations can go as high as 100–10,000 mg a day. Vitamin C is generally considered nontoxic, even in massive doses.

Nutrient	Functions and Benefits	Food Sources	DRI (Daily Recommended Intake)
Folic acid Vitamin B_9 Folate, folacin	A co-worker of vitamin B_{12}, folic acid is essential for red blood cell formation, and production of RNA and DNA. Folic acid aids with protein metabolism. Adequate amounts of this nutrient in the first stage of pregnancy can help prevent neural tube birth defects. Deficiencies include anemia, upset stomach, skin disorders, impaired circulation, depression, and reproductive disorders.	Green leafy vegetables, broccoli (including spinach and lettuce), asparagus, lima beans, potatoes, liver, sprouts, kidney, yeast, orange juice, nuts, mushrooms, wheat germ, grain products.	.4 mg Some nutritional and medical professionals recommend 5–10 mg, especially with deficiencies, and particularly if taken with B_{12}.

Nutrient	Functions and Benefits	Food Sources	DRI (Daily Recommended Intake)
SELECTED MINERALS—natural substances from the earth or water. Plants and animals absorb them to get nutrients.			
Boron	Bone health, prevention of osteoporosis, reduces magnesium excretion.	Fruits, vegetables.	3 mg Nutrition and medical professionals suggest taking boron with a multisupplement that contains manganese, calcium, and riboflavin.

Nutrient	Functions and Benefits	Food Sources	DRI (Daily Recommended Intake)
Calcium (and phosphate)	Necessary for strong bone structure, teeth, muscle tissue. Regulates heartbeat, nerve function. Plasma levels affected by thyroid, and parathyroid glands. Essential for developing and maintaining healthy bones and teeth. Assists in blood clotting, muscle contraction, nerve transmission. Reduces risk of osteoporosis.	Green leafy vegetables, fortified orange juice, dairy products. Sardines, salmon with bones, tofu. Alcohol, soda (colas) and caffeine deplete calcium in body. You need vitamin D to make use of calcium in the body.	800–1200 mg Daily intake need varies depending on age, gender, and health. Talk with your doctor about the right dose for you.

Nutrient	Functions and Benefits	Food Sources	DRI (Daily Recommended Intake)
Chromium	Works with insulin for proper glucose metabolism and is important in cholesterol metabolism. Aids in the prevention or reversal of peripheral neuropathy and with weight loss. Deficiency results in glucose intolerance. A severe deficiency may be a contributing cause of diabetes, hardening of arteries, and heart disease.	Thyme, brewer's yeast, raw sugar and cane juice, whole grain cereals, nuts, black pepper, mushrooms, egg yolks, meat, cheese.	100–300 mcg Nutrition professionals sometimes recommend as much as 1,000 mcg.

Nutrient	Functions and Benefits	Food Sources	DRI (Daily Recommended Intake)
Copper	Supports healthy bones, muscles, nerve tissue, blood vessels, and connective tissue. Assists in iron absorption. Plays a role in pigmentation of skin, hair, and eyes. Deficiencies can include anemia, impaired respiration, loss of hair, and heart damage.	Legumes, nuts, seeds, raisins, whole grains, shellfish, shrimp, liver.	2–5 mg

Nutrient	Functions and Benefits	Food Sources	DRI (Daily Recommended Intake)
Iron	Essential for making hemoglobin in blood (carries oxygen to body cells) and myoglobin (supplies oxygen to muscles). Builds up the quality of the blood and increases resistance to disease and stress. Iron is very important for menstruating women in preventing iron-deficiency anemia. A deficiency may cause anemia, headaches, lowered resistance to disease, and shortness of breath.	Apricots (fresh or dried), peaches, bananas, prunes, raisins, turnip greens, spinach, beets and beet tops alfalfa, whole grain cereals, black molasses, walnuts, sunflower seeds, sesame seeds, whole rye, dry beans, lentils, kelp, liver, and egg yolks.	8 mg (men) 18 mg (women) Nutrition professionals sometimes recommend up to 30 mg. Discuss iron intake with your physician and nutrition professional if you have liver disease.

Nutrient	Functions and Benefits	Food Sources	DRI (Daily Recommended Intake)
Magnesium	Important for parathyroid hormone release, muscle contraction, bone formation, blood pressure control. Deficiency occurs with malabsorption/ alcoholism/ kidney disorders and may result in lowered calcium and potassium levels.	Nuts, legumes, unmilled grains, beans, green leafy vegetables, avocados, bananas.	Trace element supplements can contain 100–500 mg. Higher doses (up to 1,000 mg) may also have benefit, but more data needed. Supplementation may be problematic if you have kidney trouble; first signs of excess are low blood pressure, nausea, and vomiting.

Nutrient	Functions and Benefits	Food Sources	DRI (Daily Recommended Intake)
Manganese	Involved in the formation of bone, as well as in enzymes involved in amino acid, cholesterol, and carbohydrate metabolism.	Nuts, whole grain cereals, beans, rice, dried fruits, green leafy vegetables.	10 mg. Higher doses can interfere with iron absorption.
Molybdenum	Important in a variety of enzyme systems (e.g., oxidases). Mobilization of iron from storage, growth, and development.	Milk, beans, whole grain breads and cereals, nuts, legumes (depending on soil content).	75–250 mcg. It's not clear what the limit is, but this is generally a safe and adequate range. A high incidence of goutlike syndrome has been associated with dietary intakes of 10–15 mg/day.

Nutrient	Functions and Benefits	Food Sources	DRI (Daily Recommended Intake)
Phosphate	Bone health. See **calcium** entry. Maintains acid-base balance.	Don't supplement if you eat meat or drink sodas. Abundant in all animal foods: meat, fish, poultry, eggs, and milk.	500 mg. High consumption of phosphate may affect calcium levels.
Potassium (Electrolyte)	Along with sodium and chloride, referred to as electrolytes. Maintains fluid balance, blood pressure, cell integrity, muscle contractions, and nerve impulse transmission. Sodium/potassium ratios out of balance result in muscle and heart weakness, diarrhea.	Fruits and juices (a banana has about 450 mg), green leafy vegetables, meats.	2,000 mg. High doses are used in people with kidney disease; excessive doses can be problematic.

Nutrient	Functions and Benefits	Food Sources	DRI (Daily Recommended Intake)
Selenium	Antioxidant properties protect body tissues against oxidative damage caused by radiation, pollution, and normal body reactions. Red blood cell health. Deficiency results in growth failure, and hepatic necrosis.	Seafood, kidney, liver, selected grains. Keshan's syndrome occurs in regions with selenium-depleted soils.	600 mcg max; 200–400 mcg per day is probably more than enough; reduce dose if you get a "garlic" breath/taste.

Nutrient	Functions and Benefits	Food Sources	DRI (Daily Recommended Intake)
Zinc	Maintaining immune function; wound repair. Deficiency results in anorexia, growth retardation, lowered testosterone levels, hair loss, and impaired taste.	Meat, liver, eggs, seafood (oysters), whole grains (but the form is less absorbable).	11 mg (men) 8 mg (women) Some nutritional professionals recommend 30–150 mg, but copper should be taken in combination for high doses. Be sure to follow healthcare provider's guidance.

IU = International Units; mg = milligrams; mcg = micrograms; g = grams. (Note: 1,000 mg = 1 gram)

Healthy Steps Beginning Today

God has called His people to be a healthy people. There is no getting around the crystal-clear fact that eating a beneficial food plan that includes more fruits, vegetables, and herbs helps you become healthier, feel better about yourself, and increasingly protect yourself against disease.

The best part is that you can start today, wherever you are right now, and move at your own pace as you make positive choices.

Are you ready? Let's move into simple, practical ways to make fruits, vegetables, and herbs a vital part of everyday nutrition.

6

Top Ten Fruits for Energy, Wellness, and Power

For the Lord *thy God bringeth thee into a good land, a land of brooks of water, of fountains and depths that spring out of valleys and hills; A land of wheat, and barley, and vines, and fig trees, and pomegranates; a land of oil olive, and honey; A land wherein thou shalt eat bread without scarceness, thou shalt not lack any thing in it; a land whose stones are iron, and out of whose hills thou mayest dig brass.*

—Deuteronomy 8:7-9

Eating lots of fruit every day provides many health benefits, including nutrients vital for your health and the overall maintenance of your body. Fruits need to be a mainstay of your overall healthy diet, for they are an excellent source of many vital antioxidant nutrients and phytochemicals.

Because fruit contains natural fruit sugars, intake should be limited to no more than four servings a day. For most fruit-deficient modern diets, that is not the problem. The challenge is getting enough fruit in your diet.

Thankfully, we live in a world where so many varieties of fruit are available. The secret is to find creative ways to add these wonderful, healthy, beneficial gifts from God to everyday life.

Following are a list of the top ten fruits, along with brief facts about varieties, health benefits, selection, and shopping tips, as well as storage, preparation, and serving ideas—all to provide a quick and easy reference for adding lots of fruit to your diet.

1. Apples

Hundreds of varieties of apples are available as a result of cultivation and hybridization, but the most common include Red Delicious and Golden Delicious (both mild and sweet, great for eating fresh), McIntosh and Gala (both great for eating fresh or baking), Fuji (wonderful for baking and salads), Granny Smith (tart, great for baking), and Rome Beauty (awesome for pies and applesauce).

Health Benefits: The old proverb, an apple a day keeps the doctor away, seems to be true! Apples are a good source of potassium. They provide fiber, which helps regulate bowel movement and reduces the risk of colon cancer. Research suggests that apples can help reduce the risk of lung, prostate, and colon cancer, as well as asthma. As with many fruits, apples are rich in vitamin C and other antioxidants. Pectin, found in apples, has been shown to reduce cholesterol.

Selection and Shopping Tips: Apples, although at peak during the fall, are also generally available throughout the year. Apples, regardless of variety, should be firm, well-colored, and crisp.

Storage: Ripening begins when fruit is picked from the orchard. However, apples can be stored for approximately two weeks or longer when kept in the refrigerator (preferably in a crisper, away from vegetables). Some types of apples, including Fuji and Granny Smith, have a longer shelf life.

Preparation: Most people prefer to eat apples peeled, cored, and seeded, but most of the nutrients are in the peel. Rinse well under cold water and pat dry. To prevent browning when you slice apples, place slices in a bowl of cold water with a spoonful of lemon juice added.

Serving Ideas: Most varieties of apples are great for eating fresh. Add diced or sliced apples to salads (either fruit or vegetable). Sliced apples with your favorite cheese makes a wonderful snack. Tart apples such as Rome Beauty and Granny Smith retain texture very well during cooking. For an unusual dessert, skewer apple chunks on cinnamon sticks (available in the spice aisle in your grocery store), place in a baking dish, and bake at 350 degrees for 25 minutes.

2. Berries

Varieties of berries include strawberries, raspberries, blackberries, blueberries, mulberries, and cranberries, among many others.

Health Benefits: Most berries are rich in vitamin C, vitamin A, and fiber, as well as manganese and various B vitamins.

Selection and Shopping Tips: Most berries are available fresh from springtime until fall. Brightly colored berries with a strong scent are best. Avoid moisture in containers, which can lead to mold. Smaller berries are usually the tastiest.

Storage: Handle with care. Remove any overripe or bruised fruit and refrigerate. Most berries will last up to a week but are best when used within a few days. Do not wash until ready to use, then rinse gently and quickly in cold water (don't soak), preferably in a colander, just before eating or preparation. Berries can be frozen and used anytime.

Preparation: Remove stems and/or hull. Slice, if desired, with a sharp knife.

Serving Ideas: Add to fruit or green salads,

smoothies, or yogurt. Use as a topping for cereal, ice cream, waffles, and pancakes. Berries, whole or sliced, are great as a filling for crêpes. Nothing is better than a fruit pie or jam. Add favorite berries to any muffin mix. Best of all, berries are great eaten fresh any time of the day or night!

3. Citrus

Varieties include oranges, limes, grapefruit, lemon, and hybrids that include tangerines, mandarin oranges, tangelos, and citrons.

Health Benefits: Citrus fruits are generally loaded with vitamin C, fiber, B vitamins, potassium, folic acid, and other cancer-fighting nutrients. Citrus fruits are also recommended by many health professionals to lower cholesterol and fight viral infections. Lemon juice has also been known to relieve the pain of bee stings.

Selection and Shopping Tips: Look for citrus fruit that is firm, yet springy to the touch. It needs to be heavy for its size and well-shaped, but it doesn't have to be perfect in appearance. Flaws on the rind don't necessarily affect the taste quality. However, if the fruit is soft, flabby, wilted, or has any signs of decay, the taste may be affected.

Storage: Most citrus fruit lasts several days at room temperature but should be refrigerated to last longer, preferably in a fruit crisper drawer, for up to two or more weeks. Cut fruit, if chilled, retains almost all its nutrients for up to a week.

Preparation: Before cutting, roll citrus fruit between your palm and the countertop for a few seconds for a juicier fruit. Peel, seed, and pull segments apart, or you can slice. Grapefruit is most commonly halved and eaten out of the skin with a special grapefruit spoon.

Serving Ideas: Citrus fruit is always great eaten raw. You can also grill by sprinkling half a grapefruit with maple syrup, nutmeg, cinnamon, then grill until well heated. Serve in fruit or vegetable salads, salad dressings, sauces, or sliced over baked fish, turkey, and chicken. Colorful slices are delightful for garnishing entrées, drinks, and desserts. The colorful outer skin of some citrus fruits, known as zest, is used as a flavoring in cooking (don't use the bitter white pith).

4. Melons

Varieties include watermelon, cantaloupe, honeydew, and galia (similar in appearance to cantaloupes, developed in Israel around 1970 but grown in many southern climates, it is the only melon harvested in late summer and early fall).

Health Benefits: Melons are low in calories, excellent sources of vitamins A, B, C, and potassium. They are helpful for healthy skin and in maintaining optimum blood pressure levels (because of the potassium). Cantaloupe contains the compound adenosine, which is often used to relieve angina attacks and to keep the blood thin for patients with heart disease. Watermelon is packed with powerful antioxidants, including lycopene.

Selection and Shopping Tips: Melons picked before ripe will never reach full flavor potential. One good sign of ripeness for a watermelon or honeydew is a clean break on the stem, rather than a cut. A sweet, almost perfumelike scent is a good way to check cantaloupe and galia ripeness. Another indication for most melons is heaviness in comparison to size. Tiny freckles on the honeydew rind are a signal of sweetness, and when pressing a finger at the blossom end, honeydews should give slightly.

Storage: To aid with taste and juiciness, leave uncut melons at room temperature for a couple of days (pectin substances in the flesh softens the fruit). Most melons can then last up to five days in the refrigerator. Be sure to wrap cut melons in plastic wrap or place in an airtight container in cold storage to avoid absorbing odors from other foods.

Preparation: Wash rind carefully for sanitization. Melons can be prepared in a variety of ways—cut into halves, quarters, slices, wedges, or cubes. Remove seeds and cut away the rind. Melon balls are great for special salads and desserts.

Serving Ideas: Melons can be served as fresh fruit snacks, appetizers, salad, or dessert. Watermelon boats filled with a variety of fruits are often popular attractions at festive get-togethers. Melons can be served with ice cream, sorbet, cottage cheese, yogurt, or custard. Melon pieces wrapped in prosciutto are a familiar modern antipasto. Grilled melon slices are becoming increasingly popular as a main course. Many people like to top melons with salt, lemon or lime juice, mint, or cilantro. Another popular dessert treat is watermelon rind preserves.

5. Pears

Pears are tasty, healthy fruits related to the apple and the quince. While there are thousands of varieties of pears differing in size, color, shape, taste, and storage qualities, the main varieties include Bartlett, Bosc, Anjou, and Asian. Peak season for most pear varieties runs from August through October, but there are some varieties of pears available year round.

Health Benefits: Pears are a great source of fiber, which binds to cancer-causing chemicals in the colon, preventing those chemicals from damaging colon cells and reducing the risk of colon cancer. Pears have more pectin than apples. One pear gives you over 11 percent of your daily requirement for vitamin C and nearly 10 percent of your need for copper. Other vitamins include B and E, as well as minerals such as potassium. Pears help lower cholesterol levels and tone the intestines.

Selection and Shopping Tips: Pears are very

perishable once they are ripe. Look for pears that are firm, but not too hard, with smooth skin free of mold, soft spots, bruises, or punctures. Uniform color is not necessary—in fact, brown-speckled patches on the skin often indicates a more intense flavor.

Storage: Pears should be left at room temperature to ripen. Hasten the ripening process by placing them in a brown paper bag, turning occasionally, at room temperature. Once their skin yields to gentle pressure, they are ripe and ready to be eaten. If you will not be using pears immediately when they are ripe, place them in the refrigerator where they will stay fresh for several days. Pears should also be stored away from other strong-smelling foods, whether on the countertop or in the refrigerator, to avoid absorbing other odors.

Preparation: Always wash pears under cool water, then gently pat dry with a cloth or paper towel. The skin provides excellent fiber and nutrition, so it is best to eat the entire pear except for the stem, seeds, and core. Some people, however, prefer to peel, then core and cut into desired sections. Once you cut a pear, the fruit oxidizes rapidly and turns brown unless you soak or spray with lemon, orange, or lime juice.

Serving Ideas: Pears can be served as a fresh snack or combined with a fruit or tossed salad. Combine pears with greens and walnuts for a delicious salad. Add to cold or hot cereal. Core pears, stuff with raisins and nuts, then poach in apple juice. Purée stewed pears and season with cinnamon for dessert. You can also serve pears with goat, bleu, or gouda cheese for a treat.

6. Stone Fruits

Sometimes called drupes, these fruits are known by their outer skin and flesh which surrounds a shell or pit. Varieties of stone fruits include apricots, cherries, nectarines, peaches, and plums, as well as tasty hybrids such as Plumcots (a cross between the plum and apricot), Apriums (a cross between the apricot and plum, with the apricot being dominant), Pluots (a cross between the plum and apricot, with the plum being dominant), Peacotums (peach, apricot, plum hybrid that often tastes like a delightful fruit punch), and Grapple (created by soaking a Fuji apple in artificial grape flavoring).

Health Benefits: Stone fruits are excellent sources of vitamins A and C as well as dietary fiber and potassium. They contain phytochemicals called carotenoids, compounds that give red, orange, and yellow colors to fruits and vegetables. The powerful antioxidants lycopene and lutein, carotenoids found in most stone fruits, are considered very beneficial for preventing macular degeneration, heart disease, and cancer. Cherries have been reported useful in the treatment of gout, a type of arthritis associated with an abnormally high concentration of uric acid.

Selection and Shopping Tips: Peak time for nearly all stone fruit is summer, though you can sometimes find higher priced imports from South America or New Zealand during the off season. Growers often harvest stone fruit while underripe to avoid bruising during transit from groves to the store. Therefore, at the market, be sure to select pieces of fruit that have the color, if not the softness, of fully ripened fruit. A sweet aroma is often desirable, but often the sweetness doesn't happen until the fruit ripens. Avoid pieces that are too hard or have green spots, an often-reliable sign they were picked way too soon, or are bruised fruit.

Storage: Let stone fruit soften and ripen at room temperature for a few days for best taste. Pack unwashed fruit loosely in paper or plastic bags to minimize bruising, or place a single layer in a shallow pan. In good condition, fresh fruit will keep for up to a week. Be sure to check daily, removing any that begin to spoil. Frozen fruit, pitted or not, will often keep for up to a year. Gently rinse and dry before placing in freezer bags. The less air in the bag, the better.

Preparation: Wash gently under cool water. If nonorganic, spray with a solution of diluted additive-free soap or commercial produce wash, then rinse. Pull, pry, or cut away from the stone. Peel if desired.

Serving Ideas: Fresh stone fruit is always best and most nutritious, of course, when eaten as a snack or in fruit or tossed salad. You can also slice fresh or dried stone fruit into hot or cold cereal, as well as in pancakes or waffle batter. Fresh or dried stone fruit is the perfect addition to yogurt, sorbet, or ice cream. You can also give a distinctive Middle Eastern flavor to chicken or vegetable stew with the addition of dried and diced stone fruit. Use stone fruit instead of strawberries on shortcake. Also, you can skewer whole or halved fresh stone fruit, brush with honey, then grill until brown.

7. Tropical Fruit

Tropical fruit—including bananas, pineapples, mangos, papaya, coconut, guava, and lychee—grow on plants of all habitats. The main common characteristics include extreme health benefits and an intolerance to frost.

Health Benefits: Tropical fruit is an excellent source of vitamins A, B, C, and E, as well as potassium, fiber, manganese, copper, and folate, which are all essential to overall health. Bananas are considered one of the best sources for potassium, an essential mineral for maintaining normal blood pressure and heart function.

Selection and Shopping Tips: Each tropical fruit is different, but in general, pieces should be firm but not too hard (except coconuts, of course), bright in appearance, and free from bruises or other injuries.

Storage: Again, each tropical fruit has different

storage characteristics. In general, most can be kept at room temperature for several days or refrigerated for longer periods. Don't allow ripe fruit to go to waste, since you can peel, chop, and freeze it in plastic food storage bags to be used later or in smoothies.

Preparation: Bananas can simply be peeled, then sliced, halved, or quartered. Pineapples can be cut and peeled in a variety of ways, but most people prefer to remove the crown and the base of the fruit with a knife, then place it base side down and carefully slice off the skin, carving out any remaining "eyes" with the knife tip. Mangos, papayas, guava, and lychee should be washed, then cut lengthwise. Scoop out the seeds, peel, and cut into desired-sized pieces. Coconuts are a bit more challenging: the softest "eye" should be pierced with a skewer and the milk should be drained. Then wrap the coconut in a towel and hit with a hammer (a lot of force is required). The white, fleshy part inside can be eaten fresh or shredded for cooking.

Serving Ideas: All of the tropical fruits are wonderful either in fruit salad or with greens. All can be blended with milk (or soymilk) and ice to make thick milkshakes. All are also good as an addition to a variety of recipes, from baked goods to main dishes. Skewer chunks of tropical fruit to grill with other vegetables and meat. All (or any) of the tropical fruit can be combined in a blender and mixed with yogurt for a cold soup treat. All, especially bananas, can be added with chopped nuts and maple syrup or honey to porridge, oatmeal, or other cereal. For a delightful tropical salad or entrée, combine dices of your favorite tropical fruits with grated ginger, extra-virgin olive oil, chopped shrimp, seasoned to taste, and then serve over a bed of lettuce. For a special Southeast Asian dish, flavor rice with coconut, then serve with sliced mango (or another tropical fruit) on top as a dessert.

8. Tomatoes and Avocados

It may seem to be a surprise to see tomatoes and avocados linked together, and even more surprising to see them listed as one of the top ten groups of fruits. Truth is, both are sometimes considered vegetables, but both are botanically fruits, though the U.S. Department of Agriculture now lists tomatoes as vegetables. The U.S. Supreme Court settled the controversy in 1893 by declaring that the tomato is a vegetable, based on the popular definition that classifies vegetables by use (generally served with dinner and not dessert). However, due to the scientific definition of a fruit, the tomato remains a fruit when not dealing with U.S. tariffs.

Health Benefits: Tomatoes are an excellent source of vitamins A and C. They are also a very good source of molybdenum, potassium, manganese, dietary fiber, chromium, and vitamin B_1. In addition, tomatoes are a good source of vitamin B_6, folate, copper, niacin, vitamin B_2, magnesium, iron, pantothenic acid, phosphorous, vitamin E, protein, and especially lycopene, which has been shown to help protect against different cancers, especially when eaten with avocados, olive oil, or nuts. Avocados are a good source of vitamins B, C, E, and K, as well as fiber, folate, copper, and potassium (with 60 percent more potassium than a banana). A whole medium avocado contains approximately 55 percent of the FDA's recommended daily amount of fat.

Selection and Shopping Tips: Choose tomatoes that have a deep, rich color, indicating both a more delicious tasting tomato and a greater supply of the health-promoting phytonutrient red pigment, lycopene. Both tomatoes and avocados should be well shaped and smooth skinned with no cracks, bruises, or soft spots.

Storage: Tomatoes will keep at room temperature for up to a week, depending upon how ripe they are when purchased. Refrigerated, they will keep for up to an additional week. If underripe, place in a paper bag at room temperature to hasten the ripening process. Avocados can last several days at room temperature, then perhaps another week if refrigerated. If needed, ripen in a paper bag or a fruit basket at room temperature for a few days. As the fruit ripens, the skin will turn darker. Avocados should not be refrigerated until they are ripe. If you can only eat a portion of an avocado at a time, refrigerate the unused portion with the pit still in it in tightly fitted plastic wrap for another day or two.

Preparation: Before serving, wash tomatoes under cool running water and pat dry. If your recipe requires seeded tomatoes, cut the fruit in half horizontally and gently squeeze out the seeds and the juice. It is especially important when cooking tomatoes not to use aluminum cookware since their high acid content will interact with the metal. Avocados are another story—use a stainless steel knife to cut the avocado in half, preferably lengthwise, then gently twist the two halves in opposite directions, remove the large pit, either with a spoon or by hand, and slide a spoon or your finger inside the skin to separate the flesh from the skin. You can help prevent darkening of the avocado flesh (this happens naturally with exposure to air) by sprinkling with a little lemon juice or vinegar.

Serving Ideas: Both tomatoes and avocados are a great addition to bean and vegetable soups. Both make a great salsa dip when combined with chopped onions and chili peppers. You can purée tomatoes, cucumbers, bell peppers, and scallions together in a food processor and season with herbs and spices of your choice to make the refreshing cold soup, gazpacho. Add tomato or avocado slices to sandwiches and salads (to add color, use yellow, purple, or green tomatoes in addition to the more traditional red ones). And what can be better than mixing chopped avocados, onions, tomatoes, cilantro, lime juice, and seasonings for a rich-tasting guacamole dip!

9. Mediterranean and Subtropical Fruits

Mediterranean and subtropical fruits are mentioned often throughout the Bible as both healthy and symbolic. Varieties include grapes, dates, figs, olives, and pomegranates and are considered to be among the oldest and most widespread of the cultivated fruits. More grapes, for example, are grown worldwide than any other fruit.

Health Benefits: Mediterranean and subtropical fruits are generally filled with antioxidants, vitamins, minerals, and proteins. Grapes—red and green—contain antioxidants called flavonoids and phenols that may help keep low-density lipoprotein, or LDL (the "bad" cholesterol), from forming plaque and damaging blood vessels. Dates have been found valuable for anemia, low blood pressure, ulcers, sexual impotency, and nervous conditions. Figs are often mentioned as beneficial for anemia, asthma, gout, skin diseases, rheumatism, and circulation. Olives have historically been helpful with gall bladder, nerve, and liver disorders, as well as with strengthening body tissue. Pomegranates, excellent blood purifiers, have a cleansing and cooling effect on the system, and they are reported to be helpful in relieving liver problems, arthritis, and obesity.

Selection and Shopping Tips: Choose fruit that is well colored, fresh, and bright with green, pliable stems. Look for plump well-developed "berries" that are firmly attached to the stem. Avoid brown shriveled stems, soft, squashed berries, and stems with too many loose berries. Also avoid fruit that shows signs of leaking juice.

Storage: Most Mediterranean and subtropical fruits can be stored at room temperature, but most last much longer when stored in a plastic bag in the refrigerator. Generally do not rinse until ready to use. Most of these fruits will absorb odors from vegetables, especially onions, so avoid storage next to these items.

Preparation: All can be eaten raw, canned, frozen, cooked, or dried. The juice of grapes and pomegranates is particularly delicious and beneficial and can be blended with numerous other fruit juices to be served any time of the day.

Serving Ideas: All Mediterranean and subtropical fruits can be eaten raw or dried, used in salads or for making jam, jelly, juice, and oil. Grapes, dates, and figs are used in many places around the world as a healthful substitute for candy or as a tasty dessert, perhaps topped with honey and chopped nuts. All of these fruits are excellent toppings for salads. Olive oil is commonly used for cooking and as an ingredient for salad dressings.

10. Asian-Origin Fruits (Kiwis, Persimmons)

Native to China, kiwifruit was originally known as Yang Tao. They were brought to New Zealand from China by missionaries in the early twentieth century with the first commercial plantings occurring several decades later. In 1960, they were renamed Chinese gooseberries, then kiwifruit in honor of the New Zealand native bird. Today a number of nations produce kiwifruit commercially. Likewise, the persimmon fruit, also native to China, later spread to Korea and Japan and eventually to California and southern Europe in the mid 1800s.

Health Benefits: Both kiwis and persimmons are excellent energy sources, packed with vitamins A, C, and E, as well as potassium, magnesium, copper, and phosphorous. Persimmons also are packed with B vitamins. Many people believe that enjoying these Asian fruits each day may significantly lower your risk for blood clots and reduce the amount of fats (triglycerides) in your blood, therefore helping to protect cardiovascular health.

Selection and Shopping Tips: When selecting kiwifruit, hold them between your thumb and forefinger and gently apply pressure; those that have the sweetest taste will yield gently to pressure. Avoid very soft, shriveled, bruised, or damp spotted fruit.

Storage: Soft, vine-ripe kiwifruit do not store well. At room temperature, kiwis will only last two to four days. Refrigerated, gold kiwis will hold optimum eating condition for two weeks, while green kiwis will hold for up to four weeks. Persimmons should not be stored in the refrigerator for more than a month, but they can be kept frozen for up to six months or more. If you want either kiwis or persimmons to ripen faster, remove them from the refrigerator and let them ripen at room temperature.

Preparation: Some people use kiwis and persimmons as a healthy drink, cutting the fruit into small pieces, then steeping in hot water for a few minutes. When fully mature, both fruits are deliciously sweet and can be eaten fresh, dried, raw, or cooked (if, however, your lips pucker because of the bitter taste when you eat a persimmon, it is likely unripe). Both kiwis and persimmons can either be peeled and dried whole or cut into slices (peeled or unpeeled) and dried that way. When firm, astringent persimmons are peeled and dried whole, they lose all their astringency and develop a sweet, datelike consistency.

Serving Ideas: When eaten fresh, both kiwis and persimmons are usually peeled and cut into quarters or eaten whole like an apple. Both fruits add a dramatic tropical flair to any fruit salad. Mix sliced kiwifruit, persimmons, oranges, and pineapples together to make chutney that can be served as an accompaniment to chicken or fish. Or blend kiwifruit or persimmons with cantaloupe in a food processor to make a chilled soup. For a creamier consistency, blend in yogurt with the fruit mixture.

Fruit—Great for Your Health

There you have them, the top ten fruits. As you make the transition from the typical modern diet of very few fruits to a healthier lifestyle that should include at least two cups or two to four servings of fruit each day, it is important to remember that the reasons for eating more fruit every day are clearcut: people who eat more fruits and vegetables as part of an overall healthy lifestyle generally reduce the risk of many chronic diseases and have healthier bodies.

7

Top Ten Vegetables for Energy, Wellness, and Power

Better a meal of vegetables where there is love than a fattened calf with hatred.
—Proverbs 15:17, NIV

Mama was right when she insisted, "Eat your vegetables!" Governmental and nutritional studies agree with her. Eating vegetables provides health benefits in so many ways, both in providing nutrients vital for health and maintenance of your body and helping to reduce the risk for so many diseases—cardiovascular, cancer, heart, diabetes, bone loss, high blood pressure, and more.

Most vegetables are naturally low in fat and calories. They provide the widest range of nutrients and phytochemicals, especially fiber and carotenes, of any food class. None have cholesterol, though sauces or seasonings may add fat, calories, or cholesterol. In addition, vegetables are important sources of many nutrients that keep you strong and healthy, notably potassium, dietary fiber, folate (folic acid), as well as vitamins A, E, and C.

Most nutritionists agree that you need at least 2 1/2 cups or 3–5 servings of veggies each day. Any vegetable or 100 percent vegetable juice counts as a member of the vegetable group. Vegetables may be raw or cooked; fresh, frozen, canned, or dried/dehydrated; and may be whole, cut up, or mashed, as explained throughout this chapter and the remainder of the book. The secret, as with fruits and herbs, is to begin adding a few of these nutritious, natural gifts to your diet as you learn more about the variety and preparation.

There are many ways to organize vegetables into different subgroups, based on their nutrient content and how they are grown. Following are the top ten vegetables, along with brief facts about varieties, health benefits, selection and shopping tips, as well as storage, preparation, and serving ideas—all to provide a quick and easy reference for adding lots of vegetable to your diet.

1. Western Brassicas

This group of vegetables includes broccoli, Brussels sprouts, cabbage, and cauliflower. All are members of the cruciferous (cabbage) family. Members of this vegetable grouping, along with potatoes, have sometimes been maligned throughout history as a last-resort vegetable during the worst of times (including famine and war), but these vegetables are worth a new look (and taste) as you seek to add colorful variety and healthy value to your table. Dr. Don Colbert recommends eating one of the cruciferous vegetables at least three to six times each week.[1]

Health Benefits: Western brassicas are excellent sources of vitamins C and A, as well as fiber and folate (folic acid).

Selection and Shopping Tips: Generally, broccoli,

Brussels sprouts, cabbage, and cauliflower are available most of the year, with peak season from midautumn through midspring. Each head will last longer if you choose produce that is firm, fresh looking, and without brown spots. Size doesn't affect quality of taste.

Storage: You can keep most Western brassicas refrigerated in the crisper section of the refrigerator, unwashed and in plastic tubs or wrapped in plastic for at least three to four days, perhaps up to ten days.

Preparation: Generally, depending upon final use, trim ends and peel the stalks (or in the case of cabbage, cut or peel away from the core. Usually it is best to rinse in cold water before peeling, cutting, or cooking.

Serving Ideas: Western brassicas are great steamed (perhaps topped with a creamy cheese or herb sauce), sautéed with onions and dried cherries, tossed raw or cooked in a salad with cheddar cheese and sweet dried apples (or dried cranberries), used as a bed for spinach, broiled or baked salmon, or as a stuffing for chicken or turkey. Use any of the cabbage-family members for soups. All of the Western brassicas are great served raw in salads and vegetable appetizers. Also, many health enthusiasts enjoy these vegetables either in a juicer or blender.

2. Asian Brassicas

Bok choy, also sometimes called Chinese cabbage, has been cultivated for over six thousand years in Asia. Common name variations for bok choy (some people spell it bok choi) include pak choi, pak choy, bok choi, spoon cabbage, taisai, celery mustard, and Chinese mustard. Baby bok choy is smaller and more tender than mature bok choy. Shanghai pak choi is similar to bok choy but has pale green stalks with leaves that are just slightly darker than the stalk.

Health Benefits: Rich in vitamin C, it also contains significant amounts of nitrogen compounds (known as indoles) and fiber, both which appear to lower the risk of various forms of cancer. Bok choy is also a good source of folate. And with its deep green leaves, bok choy has more beta carotene than other cabbages and supplies considerably more calcium.

Selection and Shopping Tips: Bok choy is available year round. If you can't find it at your supermarket, look for it at any Asian market. Choose crisp, firm bok choy with no signs of wilting or damage from excess moisture. The stalks of bok choy should be thick and fleshy but firm, while the leaves should be crisp and green. Avoid bok choy with bruised or slimy spots.

Storage: Refrigerate bok choy in a plastic container or loosely closed plastic bag. Do not wash until ready to use. Refrigerate for no more than a day or two, since it is more perishable than head cabbages.

Preparation: The stalks and leaves have quite different textures, so in culinary terms, you get two vegetables for the price of one. Chop off enough of the base of the bok choy plant before washing so that stalks can be cleaned individually. Rinse stalks and leaves under running cold water using a vegetable brush for vegetables that are dirty at the base. Shake dry. To boil, cook stems in salted water for two to four minutes. To steam, allow pieces to steam for about six minutes, or until tender-crisp. To sauté, stir-fry the stalks over high heat for about six minutes and the leaves for about three minutes, until stalks are tender-crisp and leaves are just wilted.

Serving Ideas: Asian brassicas are wonderful raw, in salads, or in stir-fry dishes. Many people like the stalks raw with a dip. Both the stalks and leaves go well with flavors such as soy sauce, hot peppers, and toasted sesame oil. Small (baby) bok choy has a mild enough flavor to eat raw. The stalks resemble celery (although they are not stringy like celery), and finely shredded leaves can go into salads.

3. Leafy and Salad Vegetables

As people become more nutrition conscious, salads made of leafy vegetables such as lettuce, spinach, radicchio, and watercress naturally become an essential part of a healthy meal. Many health-conscious people eat leafy and salad vegetables as a meal. Quite simply, the main reason for the popularity of salads is the freshness of the principal ingredients. They are the most widely available of all fresh vegetables, so they are seldom canned, frozen, or dehydrated.

Health Benefits: These vegetables are filled with beta carotene and vitamin C, manganese, and folate. It is important to remember that as a general rule, the darker green the leaves, the more nutritious the salad green. Romaine and watercress, as an example, have seven to eight times as much beta carotene, and two to four times the calcium and twice the amount of potassium as the lighter colored iceberg lettuce.

Selection and Shopping Tips: Salad greens must be fresh and crisp. It is easy to spot wilted, limp, withered, and brownish greens. Lettuce and other greens should be displayed under refrigeration, or on ice as they are very perishable vegetables. Even delicate greens, such as watercress, should be crisp and darker shades of green, especially the stems. Likewise, select radicchio heads that are small and tight, with a firm, unblemished base. Leafy and salad vegetables are usually priced per head or bundle and not always by weight. To get the most bang for your buck, feel for the heaviest and most densely packed head of lettuce, for example, and weigh a couple on the produce scale. You will be surprised how a head of lettuce can vary so much in weight. A heavier head of lettuce could yield up to two or three salads more than one of the looser lighter packed heads.

Storage: Most greens keep best in a plastic bag in the refrigerator crisper. Soft-leaved lettuces do not keep as well as firm greens. At most, generally buy only enough for immediate use within a couple of days. Also, avoid storing greens near fruits, such as apples or bananas, which give off ethylene gas as they ripen, thereby causing brown spots on the vegetables and rapid spoiling.

Preparation: Greens must be washed, trimmed, and often cored before you put them in the salad bowl. Twist off the stem and separate the leaves before washing. Prepare only the amount of greens that you plan to use at one sitting. Many people prefer a salad spinner to dry the leaves more quickly, especially if they prefer dry leaves to allow salad dressing to adhere more thoroughly. The big debate about leafy salad vegetables is whether you should tear leaves by hand or cut them with a knife—either way is good and has its own proponents.

Serving Ideas: Raw salads are generally most preferred, but most salad greens can also be cooked and served as a main dish or a side dish. Try braising for 10–15 minutes in a heavy skillet, brushing with vegetable or olive oil and grilling half heads for 7–10 minutes, sautéing with herbs or parmesan cheese for 5 minutes, or steaming for 7–13 minutes with lemon juice and herbs. Vary the greens in your salads or main dishes, and you will discover that you can enhance the nutritional content while varying the tastes and textures.

4. Fruiting and Flowering Vegetables

Few would argue that the purple eggplant, green cucumbers, yellow squash (and other summer and winter squashes), orange pumpkin, and striped green zucchini are among the most beautiful and unusually colored of all vegetables, so much so that some of this group, most notably the squash and pumpkin, seem to be more highly prized as ornaments or table decorations than as food. Go ahead and adorn your kitchen or dining room with these fruiting and flowering vegetables if you like, but don't forget that these attractive decorations are also nutritious and tasty to eat.

Health Benefits: Low in calories and high in water content, most fruiting and flowering vegetables do not offer major nutrients, but they are good sources of vegetable protein and fiber. Eggplants, however, are a good source of vitamins B_1, B_6, potassium, copper, magnesium, manganese, phosphorous, niacin, and folic acid. Pumpkins are especially rich, as well, in potassium, riboflavin, and vitamins C and E, as well as alpha carotene, beta carotene, and lutein. Pumpkin seeds are considered to be nutritious, as well.

Selection and Shopping Tips: Peak season for most of these vegetables is late summer to early fall, although you can get most throughout the year in stores. Avoid buying soft or wrinkled eggplant, cucumbers, squash, or zucchini—the firmer the better and the longer the vegetable will last in the refrigerator. Especially with cucumbers and pumpkins, smaller is often better.

Storage: Generally, keep all fruiting and flowering vegetables in the refrigerator crisper. Don't wash them until ready for use. Some people prefer wrapping them in plastic or storing in tubs. Most will stay fresh from four days to two weeks. Winter squash (including acorn, butternut, Hubbard, spaghetti, and turban) can be kept nonrefrigerated for one to six months, preferably away from sunlight and extreme heat or cold.

Preparation: Most fruiting and flowering vegetables can simply be washed, peeled (if desired), and sliced or chopped, depending upon the recipe. Pumpkin and other varieties of winter squash are often mashed like potatoes and eaten in bread, cake, muffin, and pie recipes. Pureed pumpkin can also be used in a variety of pies and puddings.

Serving Ideas: Serve raw, steamed, or cooked in casseroles. All can be enjoyed in soups. Peel, slice, and marinate vegetables in Italian dressing to make a perfect cold salad that lasts for days in the refrigerator. Many vegetarians and nonvegetarians enjoy all fruiting and flowering vegetables grilled or baked. And can anything taste better than pumpkin pie?

5. Peppers

Peppers generally are put into three groups—bell peppers, sweet peppers, and hot peppers. Bell peppers and sweet peppers are often grouped together. Most popular pepper varieties fall into one of these categories or is a cross between them. Different colors mean different flavors. Green bell peppers are generally stronger in taste. Yellow bell peppers are mild and sweet. Orange bell peppers are sweet with a pungent finish. Red bell peppers start with a pungent taste then get sweeter. A vast range of chili peppers (including pimiento, paprika, cayenne, jalapeños, chiltepin, tabasco peppers, and the hottest—naga and habanero) come in a variety of tastes and heats. The heat intensity of peppers is measured in Scoville units (SHU), with bell peppers at the bottom of the ranking with 0. From there you go to New Mexico green chilis at about 1,500 SHU, jalapeños at 3,000–6,000 SHU, and habaneros at 300,000 SHU. They get even hotter than that! In fact, the record for the hottest chili pepper was assigned by the *Guinness Book of Records* to the Naga Jolokia, measuring over 1,000,000 SHU!

Health Benefits: Peppers are especially high in vitamin C. In fact, their high vitamin C content can also substantially increase the uptake of iron in other ingredients, such as beans or grain, with which peppers are eaten). Peppers also contain vitamins A and B as well as calcium, iron, phosphorus, and potassium. Avoid the more potent chili peppers in case of intestinal tenderness.

Selection and Shopping Tips: Look for firm peppers. Peak season is generally summer, but you can find peppers in most food stores and markets throughout the year. Regardless of color, the vegetable should be bright with a nice shape. Avoid peppers with cracks, soft spots, bruises, or signs of shriveling. Avoid peppers with a chemical smell. Also, avoid signs of mold around the stem. When peppers (any color or variety) are priced by the pound, you can save money by choosing peppers based on the lightest weight, since these generally have less seeds. Most recipes call for the removal of seeds and often the "ribs" (see preparation tips below), so unless you are specifically planning to use the seeds, you probably don't want to pay for the heavier peppers (which can add up to 50 percent more to the price), as long as the lighter ones have the same shape and fresh appearance.

Storage: Refrigerate peppers in the crisper section. Some people prefer refrigerating them inside a paper bag. Most peppers, refrigerated, will last for six to ten days.

Preparation: Wash thoroughly, especially if the peppers have been waxed. Cut off any soft, decaying spots around the stem. Cut pepper in quarters or halves, removing the seeds. You can also cut them in slivers (from stem to bottom) or rings (side to side) to add color and variety to any dish. There is much confusion about what causes such wide ranges of taste in chili peppers—ranging from mild to extremely hot. Many people believe that the heat comes from seeds, but that idea is only partially true. That heat is actually produced by capsaicinoids, natural substances that cause various intensities of burning sensations in the mouth, and these substances are found primarily in the pepper's placenta—the white "ribs" that run down the middle and along the sides of a pepper. Since the seeds are in such close contact with the ribs, they are also often hot. In the rest of the vegetable, capsaicinoids are unevenly distributed throughout the flesh, so it is likely that one part of the same pepper may be hotter or milder than another. You can reduce the amount of heat in a chili pepper by removing the ribs and seeds, but you must wear gloves while doing so.

Serving Ideas: Green bell peppers are unripe and used best for cooking purposes. Red, yellow, and orange bell peppers are more mature, therefore sweeter, and best used raw in salads. You can stuff (with meat, tuna, Spanish rice, minced vegetables, tomatoes, cabbage, carrots, or a combination of foods), roast, or use in a variety of salads, stir-fries, and casseroles. Mix all colors of peppers in a fresh salad for a beautiful, appetizing dish that can be prepared in advance. Use slivers or rings to garnish any dish.

6. Podded Vegetables

Beans, soybeans, peas, lentils, and okra were a stalwart staple of the diet dating back to Bible times and apparently grown throughout the region of Africa, Egypt, Syria, and Israel. We know from 2 Samuel 17:27-29 that when David and his army came into Mahanaim, he was brought "*beds, and basons, and earthen vessels, and wheat, and barley, and flour, and parched corn, and beans, and lentiles, and parched pulse, and honey, and butter, and sheep, and cheese of kine, for David, and for the people that were with him, to eat.*" Ezekiel 4:9 also points to the hardiness of podded vegetables: "*Take thou also unto thee wheat, and barley, and beans, and lentiles, and millet, and fitches, and put them in one vessel, and make thee bread thereof.*" Stews and breads were made with beans, proving them to be a hearty food staple for people of all classes, and they were planted over an increasingly widespread area because of the hardiness of the plants and nutrition in the bean itself.

Health Benefits: Podded vegetables contain vitamins A, B, and C as well as calcium, iron, phosphorus, and potassium. They are generally high in fiber, antioxidants, and in numerous studies related to reducing the risk of cancer. Soybeans also are high in lecithin and considered excellent for protection against cholesterol.

Selection and Shopping Tips: Most podded vegetables are available dried, fresh, or frozen, are easily digested, and one of the most nourishing and body-building foods in the world, especially the soybean. Fresh in the pod is best. Choose pods that are firm, dark green, and glossy in appearance. Avoid blemishes, wrinkling, and yellowing. Shelled beans and lentils are very perishable, so be sure to avoid signs of mold or decay.

Storage: Purchase fresh, if possible. If frozen or canned, check container date for storage length. If purchasing in bulk, store dried beans and lentils in an airtight container in a cool, dry, dark place, where they will keep up to a year.

Preparation: Shell and wash. If using dried beans, soak up to six hours in three times their volume of cold water before cooking. Soaking allows the dried beans to absorb water, which helps dissolve some of the starches that cause intenstinal discomfort. To help with digestion of the beans, always discard the water in which they were soaked. Split peas and lentils do not need to be soaked. Place in a small pot, sprinkle lightly with herbs and spices, then cover with boiling water. Allow to simmer only until tender. For okra, cut off the stems, wash, then cut into half-inch slices and cook in a saucepan, covered with water, for 10–15 minutes. Season to taste with herbs, spices, salt, butter, or vinegar.

Serving Ideas: Many people prefer the taste and nutrition of raw podded vegetables. Fresh green beans taste delicious cooked in bouillon with a sprinkling of ground black pepper and garlic powder. The leftover green beans can be frozen for future use in soups or casseroles. Podded vegetables are also popular in salads, casseroles, and as side dishes with various meats. Be sure to try edamame, or fresh (or frozen) soybeans still in the pods, which can be eaten as a snack or main vegetable dish. Boil, steam, or microwave only 3–5 minutes (don't overcook), sprinkle lightly with kosher or sea salt, then squeeze the soybean directly from the pods into your mouth with your fingers. Edamame is a major source of protein, and fun to eat!

7. Bulb and Stem Vegetables

This group includes such staples as asparagus, garlic, onion, celery, leeks, rhubarb, and shallots. Life (and food) would be pretty boring without these healthy foods and food enhancers. All are easily grown in most places around the world and are plentiful throughout the year.

Health Benefits: Bulb and stem vegetables are generally excellent sources of vitamins A, B, as well as calcium and iron.

Selection and Shopping Tips: For asparagus (white or green), look for firm, straight stalks with tops that are well formed, tightly closed, fresh looking, and with rich color. For garlic, look for good-sized, firm, heavy bulbs with big cloves and paperlike skin. For onions, pick firm, dry onions that crackle when gently pressed. For celery, look for glossy-colored, solid, well-shaped stalks that are medium to light green. For leeks, look for well-shaped, small- to medium-sized stalks with fresh-looking, green tops. For rhubarb, look for firm, fresh-looking, straight, glossy, pinkish-red and medium-thick stalks. For shallots, look for well-rounded, firm bulbs that are smooth and dry but not shriveled, spongy, or sprouting. For all, avoid limp, rubbery, blemished, spotted, or mildewed vegetables.

Storage: Except for garlic and onions (store both in a dry place away from foods or flours which may pick up the strong odors), refrigerate all unwashed bulb and stem vegetables in the crisper. Some prefer to store in a plastic or paper bag. Use within 3–4 days.

Some prefer wrapping celery tightly in aluminum foil and placing in the refrigerator crisper, saying it keeps celery weeks longer than in plastic, paper, or uncovered.

Preparation: All bulb and stem vegetables are excellent raw, steamed, boiled, broiled, grilled, and all are excellent when served with meats and vegetables as flavor enhancers. Wash well, then peel, slice, sliver, chop, or mince.

Serving Ideas: Asparagus can be tied into bundles, perhaps a dozen, then placed in a pot of water with the tips up and the stalk ends in the water. Add only enough water to cover the stalks, but not the tips, and cook for 10 minutes. Serve with butter and pepper (or other preferred spices). All bulb and stem vegetables are delicious raw, eaten in vegetable or meat sandwiches, or served in soups and casseroles. Rhubarb is colorful and great tasting in pies, cakes, jams, puddings, salads, and sauces.

8. Root Vegetables

Carrots, turnips, potatoes, artichokes, and radishes are examples of plant roots commonly grouped as vegetables, though artichokes are actually a thistle-like plant. These generally starchy roots are excellent staple foods and usually are concentrated with energy-giving carbohydrates.

Health Benefits: Root vegetables are good sources of fiber, vitamins A, B, C, as well as magnesium, chromium, folic acid, biotin, manganese, niacin, phosphorous, riboflavin, and potassium. In addition, leaves of root vegetables such as carrots, turnips, and radishes are great sources of nutrition. The leaves of a radish, for example, contain almost six times the vitamin C of the root. Potatoes are also a good source of pantothenic acid.

Selection and Shopping Tips: All root vegetables should generally be firm, compact, and heavy for size. Avoid blackened or wilting leaves, as well as dark or spongy spots. Most root vegetables are available throughout the year.

Storage: Despite their sturdy appearance, most root vegetables are very perishable. Potatoes and turnips will last longer if stored in a cool, dry place. Other root vegetables should be refrigerated in the crisper section where they will last 4–6 days or longer. Keep carrots and radishes fresher and make them last longer by removing them from the bags they came in and placing them in a looser plastic bag with holes in it. You can use a plastic mesh bag or poke your own holes in a plastic bag. Then place the carrots and radishes in the crisper drawer. Root vegetables generally last longer in the crisper if leaves are removed.

Preparation: Wash thoroughly before peeling, slicing, chopping, grating, or mincing. Artichokes take extra preparation. After rinsing, cut off the artichoke's inedible leaves at the top (perhaps an inch), then trim the tops of all the leaves that remain with kitchen shears and place the entire artichoke into a bowl of cold water with a tablespoon of either vinegar or lemon juice until you are ready to steam, bake, or boil them.

Serving Ideas: All root vegetables are superb when served raw, steamed, boiled, broiled, or grilled. There are a myriad of other uses, as well. All stir-fry nicely and do well in homemade soups. Cook for flavorful fresh side dishes. Grate carrots into a wonderful carrot-raisin salad. Artichoke leaves and hearts are excellent when served with a dish of raw or steamed vegetables, but be careful to steam only long enough for softening. For a festive, tangy salad, combine root vegetables such as chopped carrots, radishes, and turnips with sliced oranges, marinated with a little lemon juice and honey for a half hour before serving. All are tasty in casseroles, stir-fries, soups, roasted whole, or even pickled.

9. Corn

There are many varieties of corn, including sweet and baby corn. It is often called maize in Native American cultures. Corn comes in a variety of colors, as well, from the whitest white to the most golden gold, and even in a variety of blues, reds, and oranges. Technically, corn is a grain, but many people include it in the vegetable family. Well-known corn products include grits and polenta (cooked cornmeal).

Health Benefits: Fresh corn contains many nutrients, including vitamins A, B_1, B_5, C, and E, as well as calcium, folic acid, iron, magnesium, and phosphorus. It is also a great source of complex carbohydrates and fiber.

Selection and Shopping Tips: Peak season is generally late summer and early fall. The best corn comes in moist green husks with a white or golden silk tassel on top. Take time to peel the corn husks from the top down while you are standing in the grocery store or market aisle. Good quality, fresh corn has full, evenly formed kernels. The coloring of the kernels should be bright and shiny. Avoid corn that looks slimy or discolored. Avoid also irregular-shaped rows of kernels or gaps with no kernels, and avoid "dented" corn, with either a slight or pronounced "dimple" at the top of the kernel. One of the best ways to test for freshness is to poke a kernel with your fingernail. Juice generally means a fresh ear of corn.

Storage: Refrigerate 2–4 days. Some prefer refrigerating in a plastic or paper bag. After a few days, the sugars begin turning to starch, the vitamins and other nutrients begin to dissipate, and the corn becomes tough and flat tasting. Don't shuck corn (keep in the husks) until right before cooking it. Corn can also be canned or blanched. Boil whole ears for 5–10 minutes, depending upon the size of the ear and freeze in plastic bags or tubs for use year around. Whole ears can be frozen for up to one year, as well.

Preparation: Wash thoroughly, taking care to remove all silks. If boiling, use caution, since the longer you boil, the more taste and nutrients you cook out. Mainly, heat the kernels enough to enjoy the natural sweetness. To grill or roast corn, remove the silks but leave the husks attached, add butter and seasoning such as dill, basil, or garlic, then put the husks back in place and put the ears on a grill.

Serving Ideas: Some people love fresh corn raw. Most, however, like it cooked, steamed, roasted, boiled, or served with other meat and vegetables in a casserole. For variety, try corn in pancakes, summer soups (chilled or hot), and easy-to-prepare salads. Combine cooked corn kernels with tomatoes, green peppers, and red kidney beans for a fresh, colorful salad.

10. Mushrooms

Okay, mushrooms aren't really vegetables. They are actually the fleshy, spore-bearing fruiting body of a fungus, typically produced above ground on soil or on its food source. Still, for the sake of this book on eating healthy, and because there are numerous types, including the most common—portobello, shiitake, reishi, maitake, button, and oyster—and because they provide wonderful tastes, textures, and healthy properties, mushrooms are included in this chapter because they are often paired, grouped, and cooked with vegetables.

Health Benefits: Mushrooms have been gathered and eaten for centuries, prized especially in Asia for their therapeutic and medicinal value, and are now produced and more popular than ever around the globe. Generally, they are great sources of vitamin C, protein, fiber, selenium, potassium, phosphorus, and iron.

Selection and Shopping Tips: Remember what your grandma told you—don't gather mushrooms in the wild if you don't know what you're looking for. Some are poisonous. Thankfully, you can gather plenty of varieties at your local grocery store, and most mushrooms that are sold in supermarkets have been commercially produced on mushroom farms and are safe because they have been grown in controlled, sterilized environments. Look for fresh mushrooms that are clean looking, plump, and firm. Avoid slimy, wet-looking, or wrinkled mushrooms.

Storage: The best way to store fresh mushrooms is to keep them unwashed and in a brown paper bag or plastic container. If you buy fresh mushrooms in a cellophane wrapped container, remove them and store them in another container (preferably a brown paper bag) in the refrigerator. Most will last a week. Dried mushrooms, refrigerated (or frozen) and kept in airtight containers, can last much longer, perhaps six months to a year.

Preparation: To retain the full flavor of mushrooms, it is best not to peel or wash them; simply wipe them with a damp cloth and gently pat dry. If absolutely necessary, mushrooms may be washed quickly but never allowed to soak in water. Varieties such as morels, which have a cap that is pitted like a honeycomb, are often cleaned with a small brush. Trim the dry, tough end of the stem. Unless a recipe calls for just caps, you can prepare the stem along with the cap. Use a sharp knife to slice, cut in halves or quarters, or chop coarsely or finely, depending upon preference. Some people prefer slicing or chopping in a food processor (slicing or wing-blade attachment), especially for recipes that require larger quantities of mushrooms.

Serving Ideas: Fresh mushrooms are superb as a garnish, side dish, or main entrée, offering an entirely new dimension of health and flavor. Mushrooms (especially shiitake) make an excellent addition to soups. Mix lightly sautéed mushrooms in ground meat or soybean burgers before forming into patties and grilling, frying, or broiling. Many people like sautéed mushrooms as a side dish, cooked with minced garlic in extra-virgin olive oil and other spices or herbs. A great vegetarian meal can include lightly sautéed mushrooms cooked with blanched soybeans, peas, or beans and thinly sliced tofu. Season to taste and serve over artichoke-based pasta (or another preferred pasta). Try roasting mushrooms in a shallow baking pan with a little vegetable or olive oil for 15–20 minutes at 450 degrees, stirring occasionally until brown. Or grill larger mushrooms (such as shiitakes or portabellas) for 5–7 minutes on each side, brushing occasionally with vegetable or olive oil. Mmmm!

Vegetables—Great for Your Health

There you have them, the top ten vegetables (and mushrooms, just for a little added variety). As you make the transition from the typical modern diet of very few vegetables to a healthier lifestyle that should include at least 2 1/2 cups or 3–5 servings of veggies every day, it is important to remember that the reasons for eating more of God's natural bounty every day are clear-cut—people who eat more fruits and vegetables as part of an overall healthy lifestyle generally reduce the risk of many chronic diseases, because vegetables provide nutrients vital for health and maintenance of your body.

Start by adding a vegetable appetizer tray or side dish to lunch and dinner. On your trips to the market, try to pick out a vegetable that you haven't eaten before. Keep fresh veggies handy for snacks. Use vegetables that add color and variety to the table. It is always best to buy fresh vegetables in season, since you will generally pay less and get peak flavor. Plan occasional meals around a vegetable main dish (perhaps stir-fry or soup), rather than always around a meat entrée. You will be surprised at how easy it can be to reach the point where you are enjoying three or more servings of vegetables every day!

8

Top Ten Herbs for Energy, Wellness, and Power

And thou shalt eat the herb of the field.

—Genesis 3:18

Herbs are mentioned four times in Genesis 1:

And God said, Let the earth bring forth grass, the herb yielding seed, and the fruit tree yielding fruit after his kind, whose seed is in itself, upon the earth: and it was so. (verse 11)

And the earth brought forth grass, and herb yielding seed after his kind, and the tree yielding fruit, whose seed was in itself, after his kind: and God saw that it was good. (verse 12)

And God said, Behold, I have given you every herb bearing seed, which is upon the face of all the earth, and every tree, in the which is the fruit of a tree yielding seed; to you it shall be for meat. (verse 29)

And to every beast of the earth, and to every fowl of the air, and to every thing that creepeth upon the earth, wherein there is life, I have given every green herb for meat: and it was so. (verse 30)

Immediately after the last mention of herbs in Genesis 1, we are told, "*And God saw every thing that he had made, and, behold, it was very good. And the evening and the morning were the sixth day*" (verse 31).

Obviously, herbs were significant then, and they should be today. It is interesting to note that at least four Hebrew words—*grasses, sprouts, spices,* and *vegetables*—can be translated as *herbs.* In today's language and cultures, the term refers to plants that are valued for a variety of things, including flavor and scent, as well as their medicinal and spiritual qualities.

For the sake of this book, we will refer to the culinary use of the term, which is much more narrow and specific: the leafy green parts of plants that are used in small amounts to provide flavor rather than substance. Herbs, in this definition, are different from spices and other parts of plants that include seeds, berries, bark, root, and fruit.

Many varieties of herbs enhance the flavors of food. The following top ten herbs are basic building blocks, but they can also be the gateway to an entirely new way of enjoying all types of foods.

1. Basil

Considered the "king of herbs" by many culinary authors and professionals, this herb is sometimes called sweet basil, tulsi, or tamil. Its meaning in Greek is "rich," which is an apt description of the herb. Grown in warm, tropical climates, it is prominently featured in cuisines around the world.

Health Benefits: Many cultures have used basil not only for food preparation, but also in baths and medicines. Basil provides fiber and protein as well as vitamins A, B, C, E, iron, magnesium, phosphorus, potassium, zinc, copper, manganese, and selenium.

Selection and Shopping Tips: Buy fresh or dried basil, available at most markets and grocery stores. Basil is also grown at home by many who love the herb's taste and fragrance.

Storage: Refrigerate fresh basil, sealed in a plastic bag (some prefer to wrap leaves in a damp paper towel) for 3–5 days. Store dried basil leaves in an airtight container, preferably in a cupboard that is cool and dry.

Preparation: Wash fresh basil thoroughly, then chop, mince, or grind to desired consistency. Dried basil leaves can be used whole, crumbled, or ground.

Serving Ideas: Basil is most commonly enjoyed fresh and in cooked recipes is generally added at the last moment, as cooking quickly destroys the flavor. Shower fresh basil liberally on pizzas, salads, pastas, and sandwiches. Dried basil isn't as pleasant tasting as fresh, but it can also be used liberally to season pastas, sauces, and soups. Many enjoy basil in omelets and meat dishes such as sausage, pork, beef, and lamb.

2. Bay Leaf

If eaten whole, bay leaves are pungent and have a sharp, bitter taste. When dried, the fragrance is herbal, slightly floral, similar in taste and smell to oregano and thyme.

Health Benefits: Bay leaves not only provide small amounts of fiber and protein when eaten, but they also contain vitamins A, B, C, and E, as well as iron, magnesium, phosphorus, potassium, zinc, copper, manganese, and selenium.

Selection and Shopping Tips: Buy fresh or dried bay leaves, available at most markets and grocery stores. Bay leaves are also grown at home by many who love the herb's taste and fragrance.

Storage: Fresh leaves are mild and do not develop their full flavor until several weeks after picking and drying.

Preparation: The leaves are most often used whole and removed before serving. Bay leaves can also be crushed (or ground) before cooking. Crushed bay leaves give off more fragrance than whole leaves.

Serving Ideas: Bay leaves, a staple in Indian, European, Mediterranean, and North American cuisines, are used in a variety of soups, stews, meat, seafood, and vegetable dishes. The leaves also are used as seasoning in classic French dishes such as bouillabaisse and bouillon. They are especially good with beef, lamb, veal, spareribs, and chicken.

3. Chives

Chives, while commonly grouped with herbs, especially in culinary terms, are actually the smallest species of the onion family. They are referred to only in the plural, since the plants grow in clumps rather than individually. Chives are a basic and common herb that should be in the cupboard of every health- and taste-conscious cook.

Health Benefits: The medical properties of chives are similar to those of garlic, though weaker, and have been shown in studies to have a beneficial effect on the circulatory system and lowering of blood pressure. Chives are rich in vitamins A and C, and contain trace amounts of sulfur and iron. As an added bonus, chives also have been known to provide insect-repelling properties that can be used in gardens to control pests.

Selection and Shopping Tips: Chives can be found fresh at most markets year round. Chives are also grown at home by many who love the herb's taste and fragrance, and they can be picked and dry-frozen without much impairment to taste for use throughout the year. Fresh or frozen is always preferred to dried, in terms of taste and fragrance.

Storage: Fresh chives should be firm, not droopy or dry. Refrigerate fresh chives, sealed in a plastic bag (some prefer to wrap in a damp paper towel) for 3–5 days. Store dried chives in an airtight container, preferably in a cupboard that is cool and dry.

Preparation: Culinary uses for chives involve shredding its leaves (straws), then using it as a condiment while whole, crushed, chopped, or minced.

Serving Ideas: Chives have a wide variety of culinary uses in casseroles, soups, and salads. They are very tasty raw (similar to onions or scallions). Many cooks use chives in omelets, pancakes, and sandwiches. They are a wonderful seasoning for meats such as poultry, beef, lamb, and fish. Fresh, colorful green chives make a delightful garnish on baked potatoes and soup.

4. Cilantro

An annual herb that is sometimes called coriander or Chinese parsley, cilantro has a distinct, sharp, and lemon-orange taste. All parts of the plant are edible, but the fresh leaves and the dried seeds are the most commonly used in cooking.

Health Benefits: This pungent herb provides trace amounts of fiber and protein, also vitamin C, as well as minerals such as calcium, iron, magnesium, phosphorus, potassium, zinc, copper, manganese, and selenium.

Selection and Shopping Tips: Select fresh-looking plants, available at most markets and grocery stores. Cilantro is also grown at home by many who love the herb's taste and fragrance.

Storage: The fresh cilantro herb is best stored in the refrigerator in airtight containers, after chopping off the roots. Some prefer to store cilantro in the refrigerator submerged in a tall glass of water. However you store this herb, remember that the leaves do not keep well and should be eaten quickly, as they lose their aroma when dried or frozen.

Preparation: Cilantro leaves are often used raw or added to the dish right before serving, especially since heat diminishes the herb's flavor quickly. Use either whole or chopped.

Serving Ideas: The fresh leaves and stems are an essential ingredient in the foods of many cultures, so feel free to use cilantro liberally in salsas, guacamole, sushi rolls, casseroles, chutneys, meat dishes, and soups. Cilantro is also great in marinades for chicken or beef, as well as curry dishes. The chopped leaves are also used as a garnish on cooked dishes.

5. Dill

A short-lived annual herb, dill is used as both a spice (dill seeds) and an herb (fresh and dried leaves). The dried leaves are sometimes called dill weed in recipes. In addition, dill oil can be extracted from the leaves, stems, and seeds of the plant and used in perfumes, soaps, and homeopathic therapies.

Health Benefits: The Roman gladiators were given food covered with dill, since the herb was believed to give extraordinary strength. In ancient Egypt it was also used as a main ingredient in a pain-killing mixture. It is considered one of the earliest medicinal herbs known in Europe, and is still widely regarded by some as one of the best therapies for stomach aches. Dill contains vitamins A, B, C, and E, as well as trace minerals including calcium, iron, magnesium, phosphorus, potassium, zinc, and manganese.

Selection and Shopping Tips: Whenever possible, choose fresh dill over the dried herb, as the fragrant flavors are much better. Fresh dill is available at markets during the summer and early fall while dried dill is available throughout the year. It is also commonly grown in windowsills or outdoors by cooks who enjoy the wonderful fragrance of the plant. Look for fresh dill leaves that are lush, green and feathery, but wilting begins almost immediately after being picked.

Storage: Store fresh dill in the refrigerator for 2–3 days. Some people prefer wrapping the leaves in a damp paper towel or placing stems in a container of water. Also, if preferred, dill leaves can be frozen, either chopped or whole, in airtight plastic containers. Some people even freeze the dill leaves in ice cube trays, submerged in water or stock, then add as desired to stews or soups.

Preparation: Wash fresh dill leaves, then chop or mince, depending upon the recipe. Dried dill can be ground or used directly from the container.

Serving Ideas: Dill can be used in a variety of dishes, including seafood (especially salmon or trout, since the flavors are very complementary), meat, poultry, dips, salad dressings, potato salads, sandwiches, vegetables, soups, stews, and chowders. Combine dill weed with plain yogurt and chopped cucumber for a delicious dip. Fresh or dried dill leaves are a beautiful garnish. Add dill to your favorite egg salad recipe. The uses are endless and delightful!

6. Mint

Mint, popular in Europe and the Mediterranean region for centuries (brought to North America aboard the Mayflower), is an herb that includes twenty-five species and hundreds of varieties. Mints are aromatic, easy to grow, have many uses, and are almost exclusively perennial. Also in the mint family are basil, oregano, rosemary, and thyme. There are several other kinds of mint, including lemon balm, marjoram, peppermint, sage, savory, and spearmint.

Health Benefits: Mints offer a wide and varied range of health benefits. Mint has been used for centuries as a medicinal herb to treat stomachaches and muscle pains, to whiten teeth and freshen breath, as a diuretic, and as an aid to digestion. Oil from mint is used today in medicines as a component of many drugs and is very popular in aromatherapy. One common use of mint (along with camphor) is a treatment for insect bites. Many people also believe the strong, sharp flavor and scent of mint can be used as a mild decongestant for respiratory illnesses such as the common cold. Not only are mint leaves considered to be good sources of vitamins A, B, and C, but mint also provides such minerals as iron, magnesium, phosphorus, potassium, zinc, copper, manganese, and selenium. And in addition to being good for you, mint plants are also beneficial in gardens and flower beds, not only for enhancing flavor (especially with tomato and pepper plants), but also for repelling insects, and providing "living mulch" ground cover. Mint leaves are often used by campers to repel mosquitoes.

Selection and Shopping Tips: Harvesting mint leaves can be done anytime. Fresh mint is usually preferred over dried mint when storage of the mint is not a problem. Select vibrant, fresh-looking, greenish-purple leaves. Avoid yellowing areas or dark spots.

Storage: Fresh mint leaves should be used immediately or stored up to a couple of days in plastic bags in a refrigerator. Some people prefer to wrap mint in a damp paper towel before bagging. Dried mint can be stored in a tightly sealed glass container up to a year.

Preparation: Carefully rinse fresh leaves, then use it whole or chopped, depending upon the recipe.

Serving Ideas: Mint leaves can be used in teas, beverages, soups, jellies, syrups, candies, ice creams, and energy shakes. Mint can be frozen in ice cube trays and used in cold teas, fruit drinks, or water as a delightful treat. Dried mint leaves should be stored in an airtight container in a cool, dark, dry area.

In Middle Eastern cuisine mint is commonly used on lamb dishes. In British cuisine, mint sauce is popular with lamb. Any fruit salad will benefit greatly by adding mint leaves. Also, use mint to enhance vegetable dishes such as green salads, marinated vegetables, broccoli, asparagus, beans, cabbage, carrots, potatoes, and corn. Mint can be a wonderful addition to cottage cheese or yogurt. Also, use mint liberally as a garnish on fruit dishes, meats, and desserts.

7. Oregano

What would European and Mediterranean food be without oregano? Amazingly, considering the fact that it is now a basic staple of cuisine throughout the world, oregano was hardly known in the United States until after World War I when GIs returning from Italy brought word of this delicious and fragrant herb back home. Its name translates as "mountain joy," which is exactly what it brings to palates in many countries today. It is similar to the herb marjoram, and they are often used interchangeably, especially since they are often both closely related herbs from the mint family.

Health Benefits: The oil from oregano is used in many places as a homeopathic antibacterial agent to treat infections. Oregano is an excellent source of vitamins A, B, C, and E, as well as iron, manganese, and dietary fiber. In addition, oregano is a good source of calcium, magnesium, phosphorus, potassium, zinc, copper, selenium, and omega-3 fatty acids.

Selection and Shopping Tips: Fresh oregano is superior in flavor and health benefits to dried. Look for vibrant green leaves with no yellowing or dark spots.

Storage: Refrigerate fresh oregano for 5–7 days. Many prefer to wrap oregano in damp paper towels, but it can be frozen whole or chopped. Dried oregano, available any time of the year, can be stored in tightly sealed containers (preferably glass) for up to six months.

Preparation: Wash leaves under running water or swish in a bowl of water. Use it whole or chopped, depending upon the recipe. Generally, since heat can destroy the aroma and delicate flavors of oregano, the herb is best added toward the end of the cooking process.

Serving Ideas: Two favorites—pizza and spaghetti! Oregano is great as a cooked ingredient in these two meals, but it also makes a great garnish. Omelets are great with this herb. Put a few sprigs of oregano in a dish of extra-virgin olive oil, then dip fresh bread into the mixture. Better yet, dip fresh garlic bread (sprinkled with oregano) in the oil mixture. Add oregano to salad dressings, meat, poultry, and fish. For a unique-tasting and healthy dish, sauté oregano with mushrooms and onions.

8. Parsley

Considered to be one of the world's most popular herbs, parsley is used so commonly for garnishing dishes that many people forget how superb it can be as an ingredient in recipes or eaten raw. Actually, parsley is a member of the same vegetable family as carrots and celery, but since it is most often used as a garnish, it is used in a culinary sense as an herb.

Health Benefits: Used as a medicine long before it was consumed as a food, parsley is extremely rich in nutrients. It is high in chlorophyll and carotenes. Parsley is also a good source of vitamins A, B, C and E, as well as phosphorus, potassium, zinc, copper, manganese, and selenium. Studies have shown parsley to be effective in inhibiting cancer, and this versatile plant is also a powerful source of folic acid, one of the most important B vitamins that has been shown to be effective in promoting cardiovascular health. Herbalists have long made use of parsley's diuretic effect to control the body's water levels, which some believe can help lower high blood pressure. Many also use this plant to improve digestion. As an added bonus, parsley also has the ability to help cleanse your palate between courses and even freshen your breath at the end of a meal (and all this time you thought restaurants used it solely as a colorful garnish).

Selection and Shopping Tips: Available all year in most supermarkets, it is also a popular windowsill and herb garden plant since it is a biennial that will come up year after year once it is established in your garden. Dried parsley can also be purchased, but it is not preferred by most cooks, since it sometimes has a tinny or metallic taste. Choose fresh parsley bunches that are deep green, fresh looking, and crisp. Avoid bunches that have leaves that are wilted or yellowish.

Storage: Refrigerate fresh parsley in a plastic bag. If slightly wilted, sprinkle lightly with water before storing in the refrigerator. Some people prefer refrigerating parsley in a tall glass of water. Chilled parsley will remain fresh 2–3 days.

Preparation: Fresh parsley should be washed right before using since it is highly fragile. Place it in a bowl of cold water and swish it around. Use whole or chopped. Both leaves and stems may be used, depending upon the recipe.

Serving Ideas: With the increasing popularity of juicers, parsley is considered one of the best ingredients to add to "energy elixirs." Parsley is also a common ingredient in the Mediterranean dish called tabbouli (or tabbouleh). Use liberally in salads, vegetable sautés, soups, stews, and sauces. Many people also especially enjoy adding parsley before grilling fish. It makes a wonderful addition to fresh breads and to butter. For a festive salad, combine parsley with sliced or sectioned oranges, cherry tomatoes, pumpkin seeds, cranberries, and fennel.

9. Rosemary

Some people call rosemary the "evergreen" herb. It does look like pine-tree needles and has a piney fragrance. Indeed, it grows on a small evergreen shrub and is related to the mint family. Its hearty aroma, memorable flavor, and special health benefits are all reasons to make rosemary a staple in your kitchen.

Health Benefits: Historically, many cultures have believed that rosemary helps with memory. For many reasons, it has been held in reverence. Modern studies have shown it to be a good source of antioxidants and flavonoids that stimulate the immune system, increase circulation, and improve digestion. This versatile herb is a good source of fiber, vitamins A, B, C, and E, as well as minerals such as iron, magnesium, phosphorus, potassium, zinc, copper, manganese, and selenium. Rosemary has also been shown to contribute toward increasing blood flow to the head and brain, so perhaps ancient cultures were right!

Selection and Shopping Tips: As an evergreen, rosemary is available throughout the year. Whenever possible, choose fresh rosemary over the dried herb for both enhanced flavor and fragrance. Fresh rosemary should be deep green or sage green in color. Pick fresh-looking plants that are free from dark spots or yellowed areas.

Storage: Refrigerate fresh rosemary for up to a week. Some prefer to wrap it in a damp paper towel. Dried rosemary can last up to three months if stored in airtight glass containers.

Preparation: Rinse under cool water, then pat dry. Most recipes ask for the leaves only, and these can easily be removed from the stem. You can also use the entire sprig, leaf and stem together, while cooking soups, meat dishes, or stews, then remove the entire sprig before serving.

Serving Ideas: Because it is a strong, pungent herb, use rosemary sparingly in most dishes. It is ideal for meats, poultry, stuffing, herb breads, green salads, vegetable dishes, and marinades. It is also a nice addition to tomato sauces, deviled eggs, omelets, soups, and breads. For a delightful dipping sauce for bread, purée fresh rosemary leaves with extra-virgin olive oil.

10. Thyme

Thyme is a small, evergreen shrub and member of the mint family that packs a penetrating fragrance. Thyme leaves are delicate with a greenish-gray upper leaf and whitish underside.

Health Benefits: For centuries thyme has been used in natural medicine to help with coughs, bronchitis, chest congestion, and other respiratory problems. Today's research also shows that this herb may help with brain function. Thyme is a good source of vitamins A, B, C, and E, and in addition to being a good source of calcium and fiber, it provides trace minerals such as iron, magnesium, phosphorus, potassium, zinc, copper, manganese, and selenium.

Selection and Shopping Tips: Both fresh and dried thyme are available throughout the year in most supermarkets. Fresh thyme is usually much more flavorful than the dried herb. Fresh thyme leaves should be a vibrant greenish-gray color and free from both yellowing and dark spots.

Storage: Refrigerate fresh thyme for up to a week. Some prefer wrapping it in a damp paper towel. Dried thyme, kept in a tightly sealed glass container, should keep fresh up to six months.

Preparation: Wash fresh leaves before using. Dried thyme often has less flavor than fresh, so you may want to add slightly more dried, depending upon preference. Both fresh and dried thyme should be added toward the end of the cooking process to avoid loss of flavor.

Serving Ideas: The culinary world often prefers what the French call *bouquet garni*—fresh sprigs of thyme, parsley, and bay leaves that are tied into a bundle with twine or a string (or sometimes placed into a net, sachet, or tea strainer) and used together as a seasoning blend for soups, stews, stocks, sauces, and such *entrées magnifiques* as Beef Bourguignon or *pot-au-feu* (French for "pot on the fire," a favorite French boiled dinner. For the less adventuresome, add thyme to all kinds of bean dishes or fish (grilled, baked, or poached). Vegetable side dishes such as beets, tomatoes, mushrooms, potatoes, onions, and artichokes can benefit greatly from thyme, added sparingly. For a vegetarian treat, cook thyme with a basic vegetable broth and sliced or cubed tofu.

Herbs—Great for Your Health and Your Lifestyle

There you have them, the top ten herbs for wellness, health, and power (not to mention taste!). There are many, many more that you should begin to use—from fennel to lemongrass, sage, savory, and tarragon. As you learn to experiment with a wider variety of herbs, you may want to consider growing your own herb garden. This can be done on windowsills in the smallest apartment or in pots, boxes, or raised beds in the largest country estate.

Herbs are relatively easy to grow. Once planted in the proper soil, they flourish with little care. They winter well, are drought tolerant, and most come back year after year. They are naturally beautiful and aromatic, and what could taste better than seasonings harvested from your own garden?

The development of both culinary tastes and homeopathic medicine continues to encourage people of all cultures, ages, and economic levels to grow and use fresh herbs. You can, too!

What a blessing from God: "*For the earth which drinketh in the rain that cometh oft upon it, and bringeth forth herbs meet for them by whom it is dressed, receiveth blessing from God*" (Hebrews 6:7).

Be open to the wonderful benefits of herbs as you seek to nurture a healthier lifestyle. Try herbs you've never tried before as you experiment with recipes with those exot ic-sounding names. You may surprise yourself at how proficient you become in using these healthy, tasty, and significant treats that God provided as far back as the Garden of Eden!

9

Top Ten Breakfast Hints for Eating More Fruits, Vegetables, and Herbs

Cause me to hear thy lovingkindness in the morning; for in thee do I trust: cause me to know the way wherein I should walk; for I lift up my soul unto thee.

—Psalm 143:8

Today's typical household looks like a whirlwind in the morning—rushing to shower, get ready for work, rushing out the door, then driving to school or work to actually begin the day. There is little time for breakfast. It is easy to grab a pastry, calorie-filled fast-food meal, or simply down a cup or two (or three!) of coffee.

None of those options is the best way to start your day, but it is a dilemma that so many people face. There doesn't seem to be much of a place for healthy food, which can leave you filled with calories and carbs or with an empty stomach. Either way, your sugar levels may be very high or low, which often leads to more bad choices during the remainder of the morning as you ride the roller-coaster blood-sugar ride that too many modern people know too well.

Truthfully, even in our rush-rush world, there are many healthy breakfast options. Here are ten to get you started:

1. Get up a few minutes early and make a nutritious fresh-fruit breakfast drink. Try a smoothie made in the blender with yogurt, sliced fruit (strawberries, peaches, pineapples, or blueberries), low-fat milk (or soymilk), and a dab of honey. Add a few cubes of ice if you want a "slushier" taste. Throw in some soy protein power if you desire.

2. Try topping your favorite cereal (preferably oatmeal or a whole-grain, high-fiber variety, rather than the typical sugar-filled ones), with sliced or chopped fresh fruit (bananas, peaches, strawberries, kiwi, or any type of berry). Add a little cinnamon and honey instead of sugar. Throw in some ground flaxseed and sliced almonds. Instead of mostly empty calories, you are getting power foods that are filled with fiber, nutrients, protein, and taste. Best of all, preparation time can be as short as a few minutes once you get familiar with the routine.

3. Skip the cereal completely and serve yourself a power-packed bowl of mixed fresh fruit for breakfast. A good combination can include pineapple chunks, seedless grapes, banana slices, honeydew and cantaloupe balls, diced apples, and orange wedges, plus some canned no-sugar-added fruit cocktail, which adds juice. Also, squeeze a little lemon into the mix, which adds ascorbic acid to keep the fruit from browning. This healthy breakfast can be prepared the night before and refrigerated for serving quickly in the morning. Take a container with you to work or school, as well, for a healthy snack later in the morning.

4. If you enjoy scrambled eggs, add a tasty variety

of onions, green peppers, scallions, other veggies, and your preferred breakfast meat to make your own version of a Denver omelet. Throw in light soy sauce, hot sauce, garlic powder, and perhaps a little oregano or chives. For a healthier alternative, scramble only the egg whites with the blend of veggies and flavorings. Or skip the scrambled eggs and meat altogether, stir-fry the vegetables and flavorings with sliced or chopped tofu in a little extra-virgin olive oil. Eat with a piece of whole-grain toast. It only takes 5–10 minutes, but the delicious aroma, taste, and nutrition will stay with you throughout the morning.

5. Do you crave waffles or pancakes but want to avoid the typical butter-and-syrup version and the inevitable midmorning sugar blahs? Try waffles or pancakes topped with fresh sliced fruit such as blueberries, sliced strawberries, peaches, or bananas. Better yet, try a combination of fruits. By foregoing the butter and syrup, you avoid 200–900 empty calories (depending upon how much you use). The fruit adds an appetizing appeal as well as a nutritious alternative to syrup.

6. Add chopped pears, grated ginger, and honey to millet porridge (or any hot, whole-grain cereal) for a pungently sweet breakfast treat.

7. Make a quick breakfast pizza using a tortilla (flour or corn) with a little leftover pizza or spaghetti sauce, covered with chopped or sliced onions, peppers, mushrooms, oregano, and parsley. Top with thin slices of cheese then place for a few minutes in a broiler or toaster oven. It's quick, nutritious, and you are starting off the day with a full serving of veggies.

8. Try topping low-fat cottage cheese with fresh

fruit—apples, citrus, berries, bananas, or melon balls. It is filling and can be prepared quickly.

9. There are many healthy muffin recipes that can be made in advance, then spooned into muffin pans in the morning, adding a spoonful or so of fresh fruit to each muffin before baking. Most muffins you buy at a pastry shop are filled with sugar. If you desire, you can bake the muffins the night before so they are ready for you to eat with a cup of tea or take with you to work.

10. Make a fruit frappé. Save leftover fruit juices from canned fruit used in other recipes, then add fresh, canned, or frozen fruit in a container until you have 3–4 cups. Freeze in sectioned ice cube trays. When you are ready to make your frappé, put as many cubes as desired into a blender and mix until slushy (you can also thaw, then whip with an electric mixer). Pour into glasses and serve with a straw. If you have children (or feel like a kid yourself), this nutritious, tasty mixture can also be frozen in popsicle molds and eaten as a guilt-free breakfast, snack, or dessert.

God promised us wholeness: "*For I will restore health unto thee, and I will heal thee of thy wounds, saith the Lord*" (Jeremiah 30:17). Why not begin your journey toward restoration and healthiness through better breakfast choices?

10

Top Ten Lunch Hints for Eating More Fruits, Vegetables, and Herbs

For the LORD *thy God bringeth thee into a good land, a land of brooks of water, of fountains and depths that spring out of valleys and hills; A land of wheat, and barley, and vines, and fig trees, and pomegranates; a land of oil olive, and honey; A land wherein thou shalt eat bread without scarceness, thou shalt not lack any thing in it.... When thou hast eaten and art full, then thou shalt bless the* LORD *thy God for the good land which he hath given thee.*

—Deuteronomy 8:7-10

Having a good lunch is important because it gives you the energy to stay alert the rest of the day. Eating a heavy (lots of meat, carbs, and sweets) lunch, on the other hand, may leave you nodding off in the middle of the afternoon.

What are some healthy alternatives that can help you add more fruits, vegetables, and herbs to your diet? Here are ten to get you started:

1. For a quick, nutritious lunch take a bag or container filled with your favorite salad. When you are ready to eat, peel and slice a pear, apple,

mandarin orange, strawberries, or other fruit. (If you prefer peeling and slicing fruit in advance, sprinkle a few drops of lemon juice, since ascorbic acid will keep fruit from browning). Add more variety and nutrition with your choice of whole or sliced walnuts, pecans, or almonds. Perhaps you prefer sunflower seeds. Toss in your favorite dressing, mixed in advance with chives, cilantro, dill, parsley, oregano, or another favorite herb. Enjoy your guilt-free lunch while your colleagues are rushing to the fast-food restaurants to chow down on their 1,200-calorie sandwich, fries, and shake meals.

2. Craving that sandwich but want to avoid the calories and carbs? Why not bring those leftover grilled veggies such as mushrooms and peppers (mixed with grilled meat or tofu, if desired), top with low-fat Swiss or mozzarella cheese, place on a whole-wheat roll or stuff in pita bread, and top with your own vinaigrette and herb (such as dill, thyme, basil, or sage) dressing? To avoid soggy bread, package or bag each part separately and assemble when you are ready to eat.

3. What child hasn't grown up with peanut butter and jelly sandwiches? For that kid in you, rediscover PB&J for lunch, only made in healthier ways. Instead of jelly, slice a banana onto the peanut butter. Use whole-grain bread instead of the white slices. Perhaps use more nutritious almond butter instead of peanut butter? How about rice cakes instead of bread?

4. Speaking of sandwiches, instead of the typical burgers or deli meats, try making your own veggie-wich. Slice your choice of onions, tomatoes, cucumbers, avocados, and peppers. Add herbs such as chives, basil, dill, or oregano. Use a low-fat salad dressing or mayonnaise. Use a soft

tortilla or pita pocket, if desired, instead of bread. Warning: Healthy veggie-wiches can be addictive!

5. Soup is always convenient and a great alternative for a quick lunch. If you desire a healthier alternative to the canned soups, prepare your own in advance (or use leftover soup from meals at home) made with your favorite vegetables and herbs. Heating is a snap in most workplaces. Don't forget the reduced-fat crackers, pretzels, or baked potato chips.

6. Speaking of soup, why not try something really different. In a blender or food processor, purée cantaloupe (or other melon) and peeled peaches (or another stone fruit such as apricots, cherries, nectarines, or plums) to make delicious cold soup. Add lemon juice and honey to taste.

7. Fruit can always be a great lunch. Try cantaloupe slices or watermelon cubes with yogurt. Top with rosemary or mint.

8. Mix diced pineapple, chili peppers, and herbs such as cilantro or oregano for an easy-to-fix salsa, then pour over sliced (cold or heated) chicken, tuna, salmon, or mahi-mahi. Plan ahead when you barbeque and prepare an extra meat or fish portion to refrigerate and use to make these quick lunches.

9. Try blending your homemade salsa with yogurt or cottage cheese.

10. There are many recipes available for ratatouille, which can be prepared in advance as a perfect healthy lunch. The word comes from *touiller*, which means to "toss food." Originally a poor farmer's dish, it was prepared in the summer with fresh summer vegetables. The original dish used

only zucchini, tomatoes, green and red peppers, onion, and garlic. The dish known today as ratatouille also includes eggplant and other herbs, and all the ingredients are sautéed in olive oil. It is often served with rice or French bread. It is healthy, filling, nutritious, and will make you the envy of everyone at your workplace.

Getting 2 cups (2–4 servings) of fruit, 2½ cups (or 3–5 servings) of vegetables, and a liberal dose of herbs becomes easier when you include them with your nutritious lunches. Take time at noon to enjoy God's bounty so you can be renewed for the rest of the day.

Good health is no accident. Planning is the key. If you eat lunch away from home, prepare ahead of time and take food with you. Dinner leftovers work great, saving you money, and they are already prepared the way you prefer the foods.

If you must eat out, try to order dishes that include plenty of vegetables and fruits. Salad bars are great if you avoid the heavy salad dressings. Also, remember that many Asian and Indian restaurants offer a wonderful variety of veggie-based dishes.

There are many ways to add more fruits, vegetables, and herbs to your eating choices. What better time than lunch?

11

Top Ten Dinner Hints for Eating More Fruits, Vegetables, and Herbs

Trust in the LORD, and do good; so shalt thou dwell in the land, and verily thou shalt be fed.

—Psalm 37:3

Remember the old saying: "Eat breakfast like a king, lunch like a prince, and dinner like a pauper."

Most people today have turned it around, saving the biggest meal for the evening. We are lethargic yet cannot sleep well because of the heaviness of the food we ate just a few hours before heading for bed. Worse, our "dinner like a king" lifestyles are increasingly leading to an epidemic in obesity and disease.

What are some healthy alternatives that can help you add more fruits, vegetables, and herbs to your eating choices for dinner, thereby reducing the desire for an overindulgence of meats, rich sauces, and desserts so late in the evening? Here are ten to get you started:

1. The most simple way is to include a green salad with your dinner every night. Add other vegetables and fruits for color and variety. Add herbs such as basil, chives, dill, and parsley to your salad dressings.

2. Another simple way is to plan some of your meals around a vegetable main dish. Vegetable stir-fry is a great entrée. Vegetable dishes and soups packed with beans, soybeans, peas, lentils, or okra are another healthy alternative to steak and potatoes. Add other foods to complement your main vegetable course.

3. When you plan a barbeque meal, instead of always thinking of meat, try grilling vegetable kabobs instead. Use chunked or thick-sliced tomatoes, mushrooms, green peppers, onions, potatoes, and even artichokes. Also, you can grill tofu (cut crosswise into slices and marinated in soy sauce, sesame oil, brown sugar, ginger, garlic, minced peppers, preferred herbs, and 1 tablespoon vegetable oil) turning it over once carefully with a spatula until grill marks appear and tofu is heated through, 2–4 minutes on each side.

4. Don't hesitate to try many different vegetables on the grill. Place a combination of diced veggies such as mushrooms, green beans, tomatoes, squash, potatoes, and zucchini on a piece of foil. Sprinkle extra-virgin olive oil, seasoning, and herbs such as cilantro, dill, garlic, rosemary, and thyme over it. Wrap the foil around the mixture to keep in the juices, then cook until tender.

5. Nothing tastes better than grilled corn on the

cob. Be sure to soak the corn (still in the husk) in cold water overnight or several hours, then pull back the husk almost to the bottom of the ear when ready to grill, remove all the silk, brush with melted butter, sprinkle parmesan cheese (if desired), then add herbs such as dill or oregano before replacing the husk over the corn ear. Grill until tender.

6. While we are on the subject of grilling, experiment with other vegetables and fruit. An increasingly popular and nutritious treat is watermelon steak. Yes, you read it correctly! It is a grilled piece of watermelon. You will be amazed at the unexpected taste. There is something about the grilling process that makes the watermelon taste so different from raw fruit. Some people compare its grilled texture to that of tuna. Others say that the browning makes it taste more like a piece of some exotic meat. Watermelon steak is definitely worth trying, and it is fun!

7. Shred carrots, pumpkin, or zucchini into meatloaf, casseroles, breads, and muffins to add color, texture, variety, and nutrition.

8. Prepare pasta sauce or lasagna with chopped vegetables such as bok choy, eggplant, squash, peppers, onions, carrots, corn, and potatoes. Be sure to add your choice of herbs such as bay leaves, garlic, parsley, and oregano. Either add the veggies to your preferred meat in the pasta sauce or lasagna or skip the meat altogether.

9. If you have a pizza craving and don't have time to make your own, most pizza places have a greater variety of veggies than ever before. Instead of pepperoni or beef (hold the anchovies!), try toppings such mushrooms, green peppers, and

onions. If you are concerned about calories and carbs, select a thin crust.

10. Use pureed, cooked vegetables such as potatoes, shallots, squash, and tomatoes to thicken stews, soups and gravies, thereby adding color, texture, flavor, and nutrients.

Making sure you reach your daily goal of eating 2 cups (2–4 servings) of fruit, 2 1/2 cups (or 3–5 servings) of vegetables, and a liberal dose of herbs is easier when you have already included these nutritional basics in breakfast and lunch.

This is important in the late afternoon or evening. You may be tired. It may seem easier to just eat the usual carbohydrate-heavy and fat-laden dinner, but it doesn't have to be that way. Getting a nutritious dinner with plenty of healthy vegetables, fruits, and herbs on the table quickly doesn't have to be a struggle. It just takes a little preparation and organization.

Start by taking a few moments each week to plan your meals, then make a shopping list. When you are at the grocery store, try to spend more time at the fruits and veggies sections than on the meat, deli, bread, and prepared-food aisles.

Above all else, try new fruits, vegetables, and herbs as often as you can. Vary your choices. Spend time learning new ways to prepare nutritious meals. Find ways to tantalize your taste buds while getting healthier!

12

Top Ten Snack and Dessert Hints for Eating More Fruits, Vegetables, and Herbs

I will restore health unto thee, and I will heal thee of thy wounds, saith the LORD.

—Jeremiah 30:17

Everybody likes snacks and desserts, don't they? In today's world, however, we have reached the point when we think these between-meal and after-meal treats need to be sugar-, carb-, and fat-laden. Far from it!

It is okay to indulge your need for comfort food. It is okay to feed that so-called sweet tooth. The secret is to do so while helping you achieve your goals of eating more nutritional foods.

Think about it, fruits and veggies were the original snack foods and desserts. We just need to learn how to replace the bad stuff with God's bounty. Best of all, these healthy alternatives are quick and easy to prepare.

Let's look at ten hints to get you started toward more nutritious snacks and desserts:

1. Instead of chips fried in cottonseed oil and laced with artificial preservatives, try raw vegetable sticks or perhaps organic popcorn topped with a little butter, dill, or parmesan cheese.

2. Instead of a candy bar with 200–500 empty calories and filled with artificial flavors, try fruit leather (comes in a variety of flavors from grape to apricot), fresh fruit, or dried fruit.

3. Instead of a carbonated soda with up to 40 grams (10 teaspoons!) of sugar, why not try a flavored soy drink or 100 percent fruit juice. As an alternative to soda, mix fruit juice with sparkling water.

4. Yes, we all scream for ice cream. It is rich. It is creamy. It is irresistible. It's no wonder that ice cream remains America's favorite snack and dessert, so much so that the United States Department of Agriculture estimates that each person in the U. S. eats an average of 23 quarts of ice cream every year! Each half cup of regular vanilla ice cream, however, means you are ingesting around 250 calories, 15 grams of fat, 25 grams of carbohydrates, and 55 milligrams of cholesterol. Do the math and see what all of that ice cream is doing to your body. A healthy alternative is a fruit and yogurt shake, made with pineapple juice, low-fat yogurt, fresh or frozen fruit (such as bananas, strawberries, pineapples, or papaya), and honey or sweetener. Blend well, add a few ice cubes if desired, and enjoy at only 100–125 calories for a 12-ounce serving.

5. A beautiful and nutritious appetizer, snack, or dessert can be made by carving out a watermelon half, (or you can even use individual orange or grapefruit rinds), then fill the melon rind with a fruit salad combination and shredded coconut.

Top with your favorite flavor of yogurt, if desired. A beautiful and tropical-looking alternative is to cut a pineapple lengthwise, leaving the top stem intact for decoration, then carving out the halves, filling with whipped yogurt as a dip for slices or chunks of your favorite fruit.

6. As a convenient take-along snack, keep prepackaged boxes of raisins handy. Or if you prefer, mix and bag your own trail-mix blend of dried fruits (apple rings, banana chips, apricots, pineapples, cranberries) with nuts, seeds, or granola.

7. Freeze vegetables (cucumber slices, carrot curls, radish slices) and sprigs of herbs (such as parsley or dill) in an ice cube tray, then add water and freeze. These colorful, attention-getting vegetable and herb ice cubes serve as a garnish when added to a glass of nutritious vegetable juice. As an alternative, freeze pieces of fruit in ice cube trays to add to fruit juices.

8. Freeze bananas (put a Popsicle or skewer stick into them before freezing, if preferred), grapes, and blueberries for a healthy nutritious snack. Serve frozen. These treats are great for children and kids at heart during hot summer days!

9. When making a cake from a mix, consider using unsweetened applesauce in place of oil for a healthier alternative. It makes a great tasting cake. Add less water than on the box directions, due to the moisture in the applesauce. You can also place slices of fruit between layers of baked cake, or top cake with sliced fruit slices for an attractive, tempting appearance.

10. A baked apple is a delicious and low-calorie dessert. Place cored and halved Red Delicious

apples (or another variety, if preferred) in a casserole or cake pan. Top each apple with a small amount of butter, cinnamon, and a pinch of brown sugar. Add apple juice to the pan, slightly covering the apple halves, then bake at 350 degrees for 25–30 minutes, or until the apples are tender. Serve warm and top with fresh thyme or a mint leaf. Baked pears are a delicious alternative.

There are unlimited ways to replace those yummy-yet-fattening snacks and desserts. Mainly, plan ahead. Keep raw fruits and vegetables on hand (be sure to sprinkle fresh fruit with lemon juice or ascorbic acid to keep from turning brown). Gradually begin clearing out your pantry and refrigerator of the traditional treats, and make sure these healthy snack and dessert alternatives are easy to spot when the munchies hit. You may be surprised at the ways your newfound desire to eat better becomes a lasting habit for you and your loved ones!

Conclusion:

Fruits, Vegetables, and Herbs Can Change Your Life!

Beloved, I wish above all things that thou mayest prosper and be in health, even as thy soul prospereth.

—3 John 2

There are so many reasons why it is important for you to add more fruits, vegetables, and herbs to your diet: helping to reduce the risk for strokes and other cardiovascular diseases, potentially lowering the risk for type 2 diabetes, protecting against certain cancers, reducing the risk of kidney and liver disease, decreasing bone density loss, and so much more.

Fruits, vegetables, and herbs are important natural sources of the nutrients that can provide a better life while offering a healthier lifestyle. What could be smarter?

God desires for us to "*prosper and be in health.*" If we follow His guidelines, He has given this promise: "*For I will restore health unto thee, and I will heal thee of thy wounds, saith the* LORD" (Jeremiah 30:17).

Discover the greatness and variety of God's bounty. Liven up your meals, snacks, and desserts as never before. Experience the short- and long-term benefits from eating better. Above all else, discover the amazing variety of fruits, vegetables, and herbs available to you for energy, wellness, and power as you serve the Lord Jesus!

Notes

Chapter 2: Fruits, Vegetables, and Herbs for Healthier Choices

1. Dawn Thorpe Jarvis, RD, LDN, "Why Are Americans So Overweight?" *Extraordinary Health*, Vol. 1, 2007, 12.
2. Jordan Rubin, "Fat Burning Treasure," *Energy Times*, September 2007, 20.
3. Wellness International Network, www.winltd.com.
4. Daniel Yee, Associated Press, March 15, 2007.
5. *ABC News*, September 6, 2007.
6. Rubin, "Fat Burning Treasure," 20.

Chapter 4: Fruits, Vegetables, and Herbs—Wellness Guidelines

1. Michael Murray, N.D. and Joseph Pizzorno, N.D., with Lara Pizzorno, *The Encyclopedia of Healing Foods* (New York: Atria Books, 2005), 3.
2. Don Colbert, *Walking in Divine Health* (Lake Mary, FL: Siloam Press, 1999), 153.
3. Colbert, 7–8.
4. Rex Russell, *What the Bible Says About Healthy Living* (Ventura, CA: Regal Books, 1996), 71.
5. www.cdc.gov and American Heart Association. Heart Disease and Stroke Statistics—2005 Update. Dallas, TX: American Heart Association; 2005.
6. Colbert, *Walking in Divine Health*, 74.
7. Paavo Airola, *How to Get Well* (Phoenix: Health Plus, 1974), 104.
8. www.diabetes.com (American Diabetes Association).
9. Airola, *How to Get Well*, 70.
10. Jemal, Murray, Ward, Samuels, Tiwari, Ghafoor, Feuer, Thun "Cancer Statistics, 2005," American Cancer Society: 2005; 55:10–30.

11. http://caonline.amcancersoc.org/cgi/content/full/55/1/10.
12. www.realage.com/NutritionCenter/.
13. Airola, *How to Get Well*, 148.

Chapter 5: Fruits, Vegetables, and Herbs—Vitamins, Minerals, and Nutritional Values

1. Reference Daily Intake (RDI), formerly known as the U.S. Recommended Daily Allowance), updated from Recommended Dietary Allowance (RDA), the average daily dietary intake level that is sufficient to meet the nutrient requirement of nearly all (97–98 percent) healthy individuals in a particular life stage and gender group.
2. B.K. Armstrong. "Absorption of vitamin B_{12} from the human colon," *American Journal of Clinical Nutritionists*, 1968; 21:298–9, and V. Messina, V. Melina, A.R. Mangels. A new food guide for North American vegetarians. *Journal of American Dieticians Association*, 2003; 103:771–5.

Chapter 7: Top Ten Vegetables for Energy, Wellness, and Power

1. Colbert, *Walking in Divine Health*, 135.

Notes

Notes

Notes

Notes

Notes

Notes